OSCES FOR DENTISTRY

Second Edition

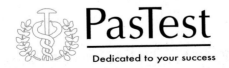

PasTest

Dedicated to your success

OSCES FOR DENTISTRY
Second Edition

Kathleen FM Fan PhD, MBBS, BDS, FDSRCS (Eng), FRCS (Ed), FRCS (OMFS)
Consultant Oral and Maxillofacial Surgeon
King's College Hospital, London / Queen Mary's Hospital, Sidcup

Judith Jones BDS, MSc, FDSRCS (Eng), PhD, FDS (OS), FHEA
Senior Clinical Lecturer / Honorary Consultant
Department of Oral Surgery, Queen Mary University of London,
Barts and The London School of Medicine and Dentistry, Institute of Dentistry

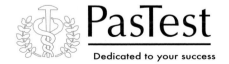

PasTest
Dedicated to your success

© 2009 PASTEST LTD
Egerton Court
Parkgate Estate
Knutsford
Cheshire
WA16 8DX

Telephone: 01565 752000

First Published 2005
Second Edition Published 2009 Reprinted 2010, 2011

ISBN: 1905635508
ISBN: 978 19056 35504

A catalogue record for this book is available from the British Library.

The information contained within this book was obtained by the author from reliable sources. However, while every effort has been make to ensure its accuracy, no responsibility for loss, damage or injury occasioned to any person acting or refraining from action as a result of information contained herein can be accepted by the publishers or author.

PasTest Revision Books and Intensive Courses

PasTest has been established in the field of postgraduate medical education since 1972, providing revision books and intensive study courses for doctors preparing for their professional examinations.

Books and courses are available for the following specialties:

MRCGP, MRCP Parts 1 and 2, MRCPCH Parts 1 and 2, MRCS, MRCOG Parts 1 and 2, DRCOG, DCH, FRCA and Dentistry.

For further details contact:

PasTest, Freepost, Knutsford, Cheshire WA16 7BR
Tel: 01565 752000   Fax: 01565 650264
www.pastest.co.uk   enquires@pastest.co.uk

Text prepared by Three Sixty Group Ltd, Brighton
Printed and bound in the UK by Page Bros Ltd, Norwich

CONTENTS

List of Contributors   vi

Preface   vii

Introduction   viii

Duties of a dentist   ix

Abbreviations   x

1   History and examination   1

2   Child dental health including orthodontics   19

3   Periodontology   59

4   Restorative dentistry and dental materials   79

5   Oral and maxillofacial surgery   121

6   Oral medicine   169

7   Oral pathology   195

8   Dental radiology   219

9   Human disease including emergencies   251

10   Drugs and therapeutics   275

11   Law and ethics   293

12   Mock OSCEs   303

Index   331

LIST OF CONTRIBUTORS

Lawrence Y-K Ching BDS, MSc, MRD, MFGDP, LDS
Specialist in Prosthodontics
Harley Street Dental Centre
London

Julia Costello BDS MSc
Clinical Demonstrator, Department of Periodontology
King's College London Dental Institute at Guy's, King's College
and St Thomas' Hospitals

Oral Pathology chapter by
Selvam Thavaraj BDS FDSRCS PhD
Specialist Registrar in Oral and Maxillofacial Pathology,
University College Hospital, London

Clinical photographs in questions 2.15 and 4.19
Courtesy of Dr Virgina Kingsmill PhD BDS FDSRCS
Lecturer, Department of Conservative Dentistry, Queen Mary
University of London, Barts and The London School of Medicine
and Dentistry, Institute of Dentistry

Clinical photographs in question 2.17
Courtesy of Mark Sayers MOrth MSc FDSRCS (Orth)
Consultant Orthodontist, Queen Mary's Hospital, Sidcup

PREFACE

Methods of examinations in clinical subjects have changed over the years. The traditional essay writing and viva examinations have been superseded in some centres by more short answer papers and practical examinations. Objective structured clinical examinations or OSCEs as they are more commonly known are becoming more popular. They provide a means of testing a wide variety of practical skills and knowledge in a standarised and structured manner. The use of clinical models has also enabled certain clinical skills to be examined without the need for patients. However some stations do require the use of standarized patients (both actual and actors), in particular assessment of communication skills, information providing and consent.

This book is meant to help students preparing to sit OSCEs in dentistry at undergraduate and postgraduate level. It includes a variety of OSCE stations and lists the things that the examiners will expect to see you carry out in order to pass that station. It shows that a correct diagnosis without the preceding steps does not always lead to a satisfactory score, and marks are awarded for things such as an introduction and empathy. It is not meant as a textbook to teach you how to perform various clinical skills but rather to provide frameworks around which most answers/tasks can be performed.

We hope that you find it useful and wish you every success in future OSCEs.

Judith Jones and Kathleen Fan

INTRODUCTION

OSCEs have been designed to allow assessment of a wide range of clinical skills, patient management and knowledge. The aim is to provide a more valid assessment of candidates in situations closer to their clinical practice. The OSCE exam is composed of a number of stations through which all the candidates rotate. The time at each station is usually 5 minutes although there may also be 10 minute stations. There are often 1 – 2 rest stations incorporated within the exam. The practical stations examine discrete clinical skills. Knowledge of history taking, examination, selection of appropriate investigations, diagnosis and treatment are all assessed and it is important to show the examiner the steps you are going through to reach your diagnosis. Some stations are patient based and you will have to perform the tasks on a patient (or an actor). Others will use mannequins and models.

We have not included a marking scheme with the stations as different examining bodies will use different schemes and sections of stations may have different weighting. However, in most cases each station has the same number of marks. So remember that even after a perceived 'bad performance' in one station it is important to move on and concentrate on the next and not dwell on the last.

Good luck!

DUTIES OF A DENTIST

Patients must be able to trust the dental profession. To justify that trust, we as a profession have a duty to maintain a good standard of practice and care.

As a member of the dental profession I will:

- make the care of my patients my first concern, treat every patient politely and considerately, and have respect for patients' dignity and privacy;

- listen to patients and respect their views, and give patients information in a way that they can understand;

- respect the right of patients to be involved fully in decisions about their care;

- make sure that my personal beliefs do not prejudice my patients' care;

- act quickly to protect patients from risks, if I have good reason to believe that I or a colleague may not be fit to practise;

- keep my professional knowledge and skills up to date and recognise the limits of my professional competence;

- be honest and trustworthy, and respect and protect confidential information;

- never discriminate unfairly against my patients or colleagues and always be prepared to justify my actions to them;

- not abuse my position as a member of the dental profession, and work with colleagues in ways which best serve patients' interests.

ABBREVIATIONS

>	greater than
<	less than
↑	increase
↓	decrease
+ve	positive
-ve	negative
μ	micro eg μm, μg
A&E	Accident and Emergency
ASA	American Society of Anaesthesiologists
ASH	Action on smoking and health
BDS	twice daily
BLS	basic life support
BM	Boehringer Mannheim (test for blood sugar)
BMI	body mass index
BPE	Basic Periodontal Examination
C/O	complaining of
CT	computed tomography
DCP	dental care professionals
DIP	distal interphalangeal
DOB	date of birth
DPT	dental panoramic tomogram
ECG	electrocardiogram
EDTA	ethylenediamine tetra-acetic acid
E/O	extra-oral
FBC	full blood count
GA	general anaesthetic
GDC	General Dental Council
GI	glass ionomer
GIC	glass ionomer cement
GIT	gastrointestinal tract
GP/GMP	General Practitioner/General Medical Practitioner
GTN	glyceryl trinitrate
HIV	human immunodeficiency virus
HO	House Officer
HPC	history of present complaint
ICP	intercuspal position
IM	intramuscular
INR	international normalised ratio
IOTN	Index of Orthodontic Need

I/O	intra-oral
IV	intravenous
IU	international units
LA	local anaesthesia
LMA	laryngeal mask airway
LP	lichen planus
MAOI	monoamine oxidase inhibitors
MCP	metacarpalphalangeal
MRI	magnetic resonance imaging
NAD	nothing abnormal detected
NHS	National Health Service
NICE	National Institute for Health and Clinical Excellence
NSAID	non-steroidal anti-inflammatory drug
OD	once a day
O/E	on examination
OH	oral hygiene
OHI	oral hygiene instruction
OM	occipitomental
OMFS	oral and maxillofacial surgery
PA	posteroanterior
PCT	Primary Care Trusts
PDH	past dental history
PIP	proximal interphalangeal
PMH	past medical history
Ppm	parts per million
PRN	as required
QDS	four times a day
RA	rheumatoid arthritis
RCP	retruded contact position
RCT	root canal treatment
Rx	treatment
SCC	squamous cell carcinoma
SH	social history
SHO	Senior House Officer
SpR	Specialist Registrar
TDS	three times a day
TMJ	temporomandibular joint
TTP	tender to percussion
U&Es	urea and electrolytes
WHO	World Health Organization

CHAPTER 1
HISTORY AND EXAMINATION

Chapter 1: Questions

OSCE Station 1.1

5 minute station

Please take a history from this 40-year-old lady who has been suffering from facial pain.

What features of the pain would lead you to suspect she was suffering from atypical facial pain?

OSCE Station 1.2
5 minute station

You are a senior house officer (SHO) in an oral and maxillofacial surgery department. This patient has been referred with pain and clicking in the temporomandibular joints (TMJs). Please examine the patient's masticatory system.

OSCE Station 1.3
10 minute station

You are an SHO in an oral and maxillofacial surgery unit. A 44-year-old lady has been referred in as she is complaining of weakness on one side of her face. Please examine the patient's cranial nerves.

OSCE Station 1.4
5 minute station

Please examine the swelling in the front of the neck in this 30-year-old woman.

OSCE Station 1.5
5 minute station

Please examine visual acuity and other eye signs in this 21-year-old man who was involved in a fight. He sustained injuries to his face and there is significant swelling of the left eye. A Snellen chart is provided.

OSCE Station 1.6
5 minute station

You are a dentist in a dental practice seeing a new patient who has come in for a check-up. Please take a medical history from this patient.

OSCE Station 1.7
5 minute station

A 24-year-old male patient has suffered from a punch to the side of the lower jaw at a party on Saturday. It is now Monday morning and he is attending A&E. You are an SHO in a maxillofacial unit. Please take a history from the patient regarding his injury.

(You are not expected to take a medical or social history as there will not be enough time.)

OSCE Station 1.8
5 minute station

After taking a comprehensive history from the fit and healthy 24-year-old patient in OSCE Station 1.7 you suspect that he has a fractured mandible. The doctors in A&E have performed a general examination and the patient does not have a head injury or any other injuries that need examining. Please examine the patient with regard to his suspected fractured mandible only.

What radiographs would you ask to be taken to demonstrate his injury?

Chapter 1: Answers

OSCE Station 1.1

1   Introduce yourself politely to the patient.

2   Chief complaint – You need to determine the patient's chief complaint, so start by asking them what the problem is or why they came to see you today. Record their complaint in their own words.

3   History of present complaint – Next you want to know all about the character and history of the pain, so ask the patient to tell you about their pain. Stick to open questions if possible. You will need to ask the patient about:

- Type/character of the pain
- Onset
- Duration of each episode
- Periodicity
- Site of pain – ask the patient to point to the area. If the area is large, ask them to point to the source of the pain
- Radiation
- Severity
- Exacerbating and relieving factors
- Associated factors
- Previous treatment
- Effect on sleep

(See Table 1.1 overleaf.)

Question	Atypical facial pain
Type/character of the pain	Varies, but often continuous, sharp, aching and throbbing
Onset	Patient will often link it to an episode of treatment Often of a chronic nature, lasting for years
Duration of each episode	Continuous
Periodicity	Continuous
Site	May migrate from one site to another Often crosses anatomical boundaries
Radiation	Will radiate and cross anatomical boundaries
Severity	Described as very severe
Exacerbating and relieving factors	Associated with stimuli that usually do not elicit pain Common analgesics have no effect
Associated factors	No local signs of inflammation
Previous treatment	Multiple previous treatments, which usually will not have relieved the pain
Effect on sleep	Patient will probably say that it prevents them sleeping, even though the pain may have been there for years
Other	No physical signs of disease

Table 1.1 Points to consider when taking a history from a patient presenting with atypical facial pain

OSCE Station 1.2

The examination starts the moment the patient walks into the surgery, with you observing them. The formal part of the examination starts after all the history has been taken. The normal rule with examination is to start with a general examination of the patient and then examine specific systems.

1   Introduce yourself politely to the patient.

2   Start with the extra-oral examination.

3   Check facial symmetry, lip competence, any gross facial/developmental abnormalities.

4   Palpate the neck nodes.

5   Palpate the left and right TMJs to determine if there is pain or tenderness to touch. The TMJs should be palpated while the patient opens their mouth slowly. This can be done by placing your fingers over the joints or in the patient's ears.

6   Any noises from the joints should be noted. Sometimes you may actually need to listen with a stethoscope, but some noises are so loud that you can hear them without it.

7   Watch the path traced by the tip of one of the lower central incisors throughout the opening and closing cycle.

8   Any association between a change in direction of movement and a noise from the joint should also be noted.

9   The TMJs should now be palpated throughout lateral and protrusive excursions.

10   Measure the maximum opening between the incisor tips (normal is around 45 mm).

11   Measure the lateral and protrusive excursions (normal is around 10 mm).

12   Palpate the muscles of mastication. The masseter and temporalis are palpated extra-orally. The lateral pterygoid can be evaluated by asking the patient to try to open their mouth

while you try to restrict the movement by placing your hand under their chin. If pain is elicited in the pre-auricular region, it is coming from the lateral pterygoid. It is also possible to gently palpate the head of the muscle up behind the tuberosity. The medial pterygoid can be palpated intra-orally along the medial aspect of the mandible.

13 Intra-oral examination:

(a) Note the teeth present and the health of the teeth.

(b) Note the pattern of tooth wear.

(c) Examine the intercuspal position (ICP) and retruded contact position (RCP).

(d) Examine group function/canine guidance in lateral excursions and protrusive movements.

(e) Note any displacements.

(f) Examine the buccal mucosa – a white line along the buccal mucosa is evidence of grinding.

Comment

Joint noises

- A click implies that there is a displaced disc that reduces to a normal position.
- Crepitus or grating noises imply degenerative changes within the joint.

Mandibular movements

- Obstruction of movement within the joint will cause the mandible to deviate on opening and closing.

OSCE Station 1.3

1   Introduce yourself politely to the patient.

2   Examine the cranial nerves.

There are 12 cranial nerves:

I – Olfactory nerve: sense of smell.

- Ask the patient if their smell is altered.
- Test with aromatic substances.

II – Optic nerve: sight.

- Ask the patient about their sight.
- Check visual acuity (see station 1.5)

III – Oculomotor nerve: motor to the external ocular muscles.

IV – Trochlear nerve: motor to the superior oblique muscle.

VI – Abducens nerve: motor to lateral rectus.

- III–VI – Test the eye movements in all directions.

V – Trigeminal nerve: sensory to facial skin and oral mucosa, motor to the muscles of mastication.

- Check all three divisions: ophthalmic, maxillary and mandibular.
- Is the sensation of the skin of the face normal over all these divisions?
- Does the patient have a corneal reflex?
- Can the patient clench her jaw muscles?

VII – Facial nerve: motor to the muscles of facial expression, sensory to the external auditory meatus, taste sensation to the tongue.

- Can the patient pout, smile, wrinkle her forehead or raise her eyebrows?
- NB: Nerve supply to the forehead is bilateral so forehead movements are not affected in upper motor neurone lesions.

VIII – Vestibulocochlear nerve: hearing and balance.
- Can the patient hear normally?
- Block one ear by pressing on the tragus and whisper a number (eg 99) and get the patient to repeat the number. Repeat the test blocking the other ear.

IX – Glossopharyngeal nerve: supplies the stylopharyngeus muscle and taste in the posterior third of tongue (injury leads to absence of gag reflex, absence or diminished).

- Ask the patient to say 'aahh' and look for deviation of the uvula and movements of the soft palate.

X – Vagus nerve: supplies structures in neck, thorax and abdomen.

- Ask the patient to say 'aahh' and look for deviation of the uvula.
- Tell the examiner that you will test the gag reflex. Although this is not reliable, and it is unpleasant for the patient.

XI – Accessory nerve: innervates sternomastoid muscle and trapezius.

- Can the patient shrug her shoulders?

XII – Hypoglossal nerve: motor to tongue muscles.

- Ask patient to protrude her tongue. Is the tongue symmetrical in movement and bulk?

OSCE Station 1.4

1   Introduce yourself politely to the patient.

2   The neck of a seated patient is observed from the front.

3   Ask the patient to swallow (offer a glass of water to the patient).

4   Stand behind the patient and palpate the thyroid gland.

5   Percuss the manubrium for retrosternal extension.

6   Auscultate for bruit.

7   Palpate the triangles of the neck and supraclavicular fossae for lymph nodes.

Perform the above examination in a fluent manner.

Comment

Lumps in the neck can be divided into benign and malignant. Alternatively, they can be classified by their location. After you have examined the patient it is important that you are able to answer the following questions:

- Is there a single lump or are there multiple lumps? Multiple lumps usually indicate lymph nodes.
- Where is the lump?
- Is the lump solid or cystic?
- Does it move with swallowing?

Malignant lumps

These can be primary, eg thyroid, or secondary (metastatic), ie lymph nodes.

Benign lumps

- Congenital: lymphangiomas, dermoid cyst, thyroglossal duct cyst, branchial fistulae
- Acquired: ranulae, laryngoceles, pharyngeal pouches
- Infective: bacterial, viral
- Neurogenous tumours: neurofibromas, carotid body tumours, glomus jugulare tumours

Neck lumps relative to location.

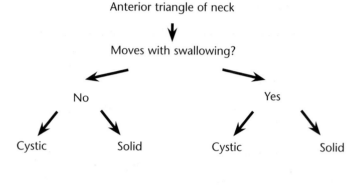

Anterior triangle of neck

↓

Moves with swallowing?

No   Yes

Cystic   Solid   Cystic   Solid

Branchial cyst	Lymph node	Thyroglossal	Thyroid gland
Cold abscess	Carotid body	duct cyst	Thyroid isthmus
Cystic hygroma*	tumour		Lymph node
	Submandibular		
	gland		
	Dermoid		

*Transilluminates

Midline structures: thyroid, thyroglossal duct cyst, thyroid isthmus and dermoid

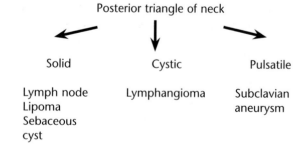

Posterior triangle of neck

Solid   Cystic   Pulsatile

Lymph node	Lymphangioma	Subclavian
Lipoma		aneurysm
Sebaceous		
cyst		

OSCE Station 1.5

1   Introduce yourself politely to the patient.

2   Demonstrate visual acuity (6/6 normal) of each eye using the Snellen chart.

3   Assess for pupillary reaction to light – direct and consensual.

4   Assess for diplopia in the nine cardinal positions – stand at least 1 m away from the patient and use a pin or your finger.

5   Inform the examiner that you would examine for vertical displacement of the globe (hypoglobus), enophthalmos and exopthalmus (proptosis).

Comment

Central vision is tested by using the set of letters on a Snellen chart. Vision is expressed as a fraction of normal (normal is 6/6). The patient is positioned 6 m from the card. Ask the patient to cover each eye in turn and tell you which is the smallest line of print that they can read comfortably. If patient is only able to read down to the 12 m line, their visual acuity is 6/12. These figures are written on each line of the chart.

(See Snellen chart overleaf.)

Pupillary reaction to light: direct constriction is mediated by the oculomotor nerve (efferent pathway) whereas indirect constriction is mediated via the optic nerve (afferent pathway).

Snellen Chart

OSCE Station 1.6

1   Introduce yourself politely to the patient.

2   Take a medical history:

- Are they generally fit and healthy?
- Have they had any problems with their heart or blood pressure?
- Have they ever had rheumatic fever?
- Have they had any problems with their chest or breathing?
- Are they allergic to any substance or drug?
- Are they allergic to penicillin?
- Are they taking any drugs or medications, whether prescribed by the doctor or not?
- Have they ever been in hospital for any operations or illnesses?
- Have they ever, or could they be suffering from:
    - Epilepsy
    - Diabetes
    - Hepatitis
    - Jaundice
    - Tuberculosis
    - Any other infections?
- Do they have any problems with bleeding, eg following tooth extraction?
- Could they be pregnant?
- Do they smoke? If so, what do they smoke, how much/ many per day, and when did they start?
- Do they drink any alcohol? If so, how much on an average week, and what do they drink?

It is also useful to ask who their general medical practitioner is and if there is anything else that they think is relevant for you to know.

OSCE Station 1.7

Any history taken from a patient follows the same routine, ie patient's complaint, history of present complaint, medical history, social history and dental history. With patients who have suffered trauma there are a few other points to consider.

1　　Introduce yourself politely to the patient.

2　　Patient's complaint – You need to ascertain their chief complaint and write it in the notes in their own words.

3　　History of present complaint – Gain as much information as possible about the injury. Therefore, you need to about:

　　(a)　Exactly how was the patient injured?
　　(b)　What was he hit with?
　　(c)　How many times was he hit?
　　(d)　What direction the blow(s) came from?
　　(e)　Did he lose consciousness, if so for how long and how has this been dealt with?
　　(f)　Was the alleged assault witnessed and if so by whom?
　　(g)　Are the police involved?
　　(h)　Was any treatment sought initially?
　　(i)　Was the patient under the influence of any substances when the injury occurred (eg alcohol or drugs)?

4　　You need to find out about the symptoms that the patient is experiencing now with respect to:

- Pain – type, character, site, onset, duration, periodicity, radiation, severity, exacerbating and relieving factors, associated factors.
- Loss of or altered function related to:
  - The mandible – movement, occlusion, speech, swallowing
  - Nerve injury – paraesthesia/anaesthesia of the trigeminal nerve
  - Bleeding from ears.

5　　You also need to find out whether the patient has shown any signs of a head injury since the time the injury occurred (although in this case the patient has been cleared by the A&E staff).

OSCE Station 1.8

Examination of all patients follows the same standard pattern. You start by doing a general examination and then move to the specific problem. The general part of the examination starts as soon as the patient moves into the room, as you are observing them. The history and the degree of trauma sustained will determine whether a whole body examination is warranted. In this question, a whole body examination has not been asked for; in fact the question asks you to concentrate on the mandibular injury alone. This is slightly artificial, as in normal practice you would be examining the whole of the facial skeleton to discount other injuries.

1   Introduce yourself politely to the patient.

2   Explain to him what you are trying to do.

Extra-oral

3   Look at the patient from directly in front and from the same level as the patient and note any asymmetry.

4   Look for any swelling, bruising, lacerations and remember to look behind the ears for bruising and for any evidence of bleeding or CSF leaking from the ears.

5   Check whether the patient has any sensory disturbance of the skin of the lower lip – this indicates damage to the inferior dental nerve.

6   Palpate the mandible gently (remember it will be uncomfortable for the patient) from the condyle to the symphysis on both sides. This will allow you to feel any step defects in the continuity of the bone and also any swelling or discomfort in a particular region(s).

7   Ask the patient to carry out mandibular movements and watch the degree of mouth opening and deviation of the mandible. Palpate the condyles while the patient is trying to carry out the mandibular movements.

CHAPTER 1
Answers

Intra-oral

8   Check for any bruising or swelling within the mouth, especially in the buccal sulci and sublingually.

9   Check for any lacerations within the mouth, especially gingival tears.

10   If there are any empty sockets, the missing teeth must be accounted for as there is always the possibility that a patient has inhaled a tooth that has been avulsed following trauma.

11   Check for any loose or fractured teeth, or fractured dentures.

12   Check the occlusal plane for any step(s).

13   Check the occlusion – presence of certain malocclusions will give you a clue about where the fracture in the mandible is, eg an anterior open bite is seen with bilateral fractured condyles.

14   Ask the patient to carry out a full range of mandibular movements and note where discomfort is felt if movement is limited.

15   It is possible to hold the mandible with two hands and check for movement across a suspected fracture. However, only do this when there is no other way to determine whether the area is fractured and only gently, as it will cause the patient pain and may turn an undisplaced fracture into a displaced fracture.

Comment

Radiographs that are commonly taken to show fractured mandibles are the panoramic and posterior–anterior mandibular radiographs. However, if a fractured condyle is suspected it may be visualised in a reverse Towne's view. Some anterior mandibular fractures may be visualised in a lower anterior occlusal view.

CHILD DENTAL HEALTH INCLUDING ORTHODONTICS

Chapter 2: Questions

OSCE Station 2.1
5 minute station

You are a dentist in general practice. A mother has brought her 6-year-old daughter to your surgery for a routine check-up. The child has had previous restorative work on her deciduous molar teeth.

Please give dietary advice to the mother and child.

Props:

- Completed 3-day diet sheet

OSCE Station 2.2
5 minute station

You are a dentist in general dental practice. A mother has brought her 2-year-old son in to see you for his first dental appointment. The mother is unsure whether she should give her son fluoride supplements, as they live in a non-fluoridated area.

Please give fluoride advice to this mother and her son and explain your reasons for the advice given.

OSCE Station 2.3
10 minute station

Please trace this cephalometric radiograph, and indicate the various cephalometric points used.

Props:

- Lateral cephalometric radiograph (see overleaf)
- Tracing paper
- Light box
- Sellotape®
- Sharp pencil.

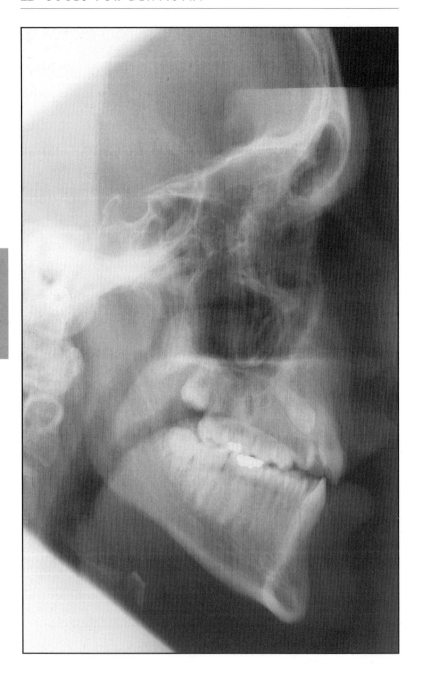

OSCE Station 2.4
5 minute station

What are the normal values for these cephalometric measurements in Caucasians ?

SNA	
SNB	
ANB	
Upper incisors to maxillary plane	
Lower incisors to mandibular plane	
Interincisal angle	
Maxillomandibular plane angle	
Lower anterior face height as a percentage of total face height	

Table 2.4a

If ANB is greater than 4° what Class of skeletal pattern will the patient have?

If ANB is less than 2° what Class of skeletal pattern will the patient have?

OSCE Station 2.5
5 minute station

A fit and healthy 15-year-old girl with a Class I skeletal pattern and Class I occlusion has attended your dental practice. She has a retained upper right primary canine. Radiographs have revealed that the permanent successor is present and impacted. The radiographs are shown overleaf. The patient and her mother wish to know what options are available to treat the problem.

a

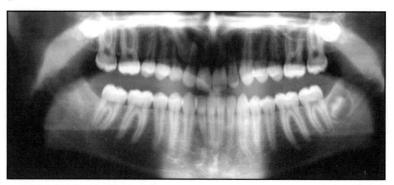

b

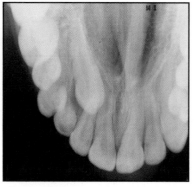

Please explain to the patient and her mother where the tooth is and the various treatment options for impacted canines.

OSCE Station 2.6
5 minute station

This 9-year-old schoolboy has delayed eruption of his upper left central incisor.

A What are the causes of unerupted central incisors?

B Radiographs show that there is a midline supernumerary tooth present. How else may supernumerary teeth present?

C Please explain to the parent accompanying the child how you would treat this?

OSCE Station 2.7
5 minute station

You are a dentist in general practice. A mother brings along her fit and healthy 3-year-old daughter who has fallen and avulsed her left upper deciduous central incisor. They have brought the avulsed tooth in a cup of milk.

A Explain your management of this. What possible complications do you need to warn the mother about?

B How would this differ if it the child was 10 years old and the tooth avulsed was the upper left permanent central incisor?

OSCE Station 2.8
5 minute station

A 13-year-old boy attends your practice after a football tackle leaves him with an injury to the right upper central incisor. You take a periapical radiograph and discover he has an apical third root fracture.

Describe your management.

OSCE Station 2.9
5 minute station

A 14-year-old girl attends your surgery with her mother after being hit in the mouth with a hockey ball during a games lesson around 45 minutes ago. Her upper right central incisor has a crown fracture.

Please explain how you would manage this case.

OSCE Station 2.10
5 minute station

Describe the procedure for a vital pulpotomy in a primary tooth.

OSCE Station 2.11
5 minute station

You are a dentist in general practice and a mother brings her 3-year-old son with rampant nursing caries (bottle caries) to see you.

What is the likely cause and how would you manage this patient in the short term and long term?

OSCE Station 2.12
5 minute station

Please construct a passive splint using this model to stabilise the upper left central incisor that has been re-implanted following avulsion.

Props:

- Study model
- Stainless-steel wire
- Dental wax

OSCE Station 2.13
5 minute station

A mother has telephoned your dental practice. Her 10-year-old daughter has fallen while roller-skating and avulsed one of her upper front teeth. She has the tooth but doesn't know what to do with it.

Please advise her as to the best course of action.

OSCE Station 2.14
5 minute station

A 7-year-old boy with a high rate of caries attends your practice with his mother. She has heard about fissure sealants and wishes to discuss the possible benefits and the procedure for placing fissure sealants on her son's teeth.

OSCE Station 2.15
10 minute station

A   You are fitting an upper removable orthodontic appliance (URA) with Adams' cribs and palatal finger springs for James. What instructions would you give him regarding wearing the appliance and its care?

B   James returns 6 weeks later to have the URA checked and adjusted. What checks would you carry out and how would you adjust his URA to become active again?

C   If James had not been wearing his appliance what factors would make you suspicious of this fact?

OSCE Station 2.16
5 minute station

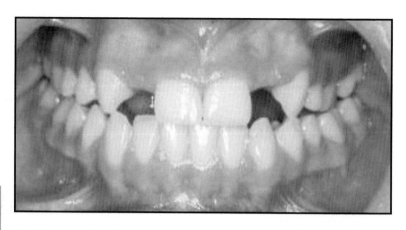

An 18-year-old patient presents at your surgery with the above dentition.

A   What appearance is shown in the above photograph?

B   What are the possible causes?

C   How would you manage this patient?

OSCE Station 2.17
10 minute station

You are a dentist working at 'Smiles Dental Practice,' 21 Borough End Road, Thamestown AB1 2CD, Tel 020 7123 4567.

A 15-year-old patient (see clinical photographs), Freddy, attends your practice with his mother who is concerned about the appearance of his teeth. Freddy says his bottom teeth are causing soreness in the roof of his mouth. He has an overjet of 8 mm. Please write an appropriate referral for an orthodontic opinion.

Patient details:
- Name – Freddy Smith
- Date of Birth – 13/8/1994
- Address – 54 Burntash Avenue, Thamestown AB18 4CD.
- Tel – 020 7123 9876

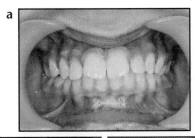

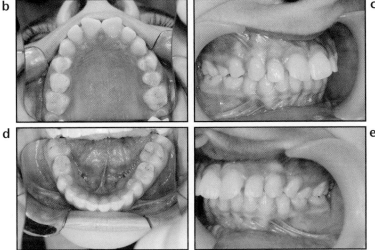

The Dental Health Component of the IOTN has five grades.
Below is a simplified version of the IOTN, which may be helpful in
writing your referral (see British Orthodontic Society website for
more information).

Grade 1

Almost perfection.

Grade 2

Minor irregularities such as:
- Slightly protruding upper front teeth
- Slightly irregular teeth
- Minor reversals of the normal relationship of upper and
  lower teeth that do not interfere with normal function.

Grade 3

Greater irregularities that usually do not need treatment for health
reasons:
- Upper front teeth that protrude less than 4 mm more
  than normal.
- Reversals of the normal relationship of upper teeth which
  only interfere with normal function to a minor degree –
  by less that 2 mm.
- Irregularity of teeth which are less than 4 mm out of line.
- Open bites of less that 4 mm.
- Deep bites with no functional problems.

Grade 4

More severe degrees of irregularities requiring treatment for
health reasons:
- Upper front teeth that protrude more than 6 mm.
- Reversals of the normal relationship of upper teeth that
  interfere with normal function – greater than 2 mm.
- Lower front teeth that protrude in front of the upper teeth
  by more than 3.5 mm.
- Irregularity of teeth that are more than 4 mm out of line.
- Fewer than the normal number of teeth (missing teeth)
  where gaps need to be closed.

- Open bites of more than 4 mm.
- Deep bites with functional problems.
- More than the normal number of teeth (supernumerary teeth).

Grade 5

Severe dental health problems:
- When teeth cannot erupt normally because of obstruction due to crowding, additional teeth or any other cause.
- A large number of missing teeth.
- Upper front teeth that protrude more than 9 mm.
- Lower front teeth that protrude in front of the upper teeth by more than 3.5 mm and where there are functional difficulties too.
- Cranio-facial anomalies such as cleft lip and palate.

Chapter 2: Answers

OSCE Station 2.1

The reason for giving dietary advice is to try to minimise dental decay. Patients may be unaware of the cariogenic foodstuffs in their diet. Diet advice needs to be appropriate for the individual, as everyone is slightly different.

1   Introduce yourself politely to the patient and mother.

2   Establish rapport with the child.

3   You would start with a diet analysis. This should be for 3–4 days and include at least one weekday.

4   Explain to the mother that she needs to record the time, the content and the amount of food and drink consumed as well as the toothbrushing times

The examiner tells you the patient/mother has a completed diet sheet.

5   The diet sheet should be checked with the patient and mother.

6   Assess nutritional value of main meals.

7   Highlight all sugar intake.

8   Highlight any between-meal snacks and assess nutritional value.

9   Keep advice short and simple, as overloading the patient and mother will be counter-productive.

10   Explain relation between sugary snacks and drinks between meals and decay.

11   Possible hints to give:

    (a) Save sweets to a special time of the week, eg Saturday morning.

(b) Eat sweets all in one go rather than spreading them out (ie a chocolate bar is less harmful than a bag of chocolates).

(c) Crisps, nuts, etc, although more dentally friendly, are very high in fat and salt and shouldn't always be substituted for sweets.

(d) Chewing gum and cheese will stimulate saliva flow and may help after eating sugary snacks, although chewing gum may not be appropriate for young children.

(e) Fizzy drinks contain large amounts of sugar.

(f) Diet fizzy drinks can cause erosion even though they are sugar-free.

13 Overall aim is to decrease sugary snacks and fizzy drinks between meals.

14 Increase the amount of fresh fruit and vegetables eaten.

OSCE Station 2.2

1 Introduce yourself politely to the patient and parent.

2 Establish rapport with the child.

3 Explain to the examiner that you would carry out a caries risk assessment for the child. This would involve assessing:

(a) Diet and sugar intake, including bottle- or breast-feeding

(b) Exposure to fluoride

(c) Motivation of the mother and family

(d) Socio-economic group

(e) Any relevant medical history

(f) *Lactobacillus* and *Streptococcus mutans* counts

4 For a low-risk child, 500 ppm fluoride toothpaste would be adequate, and this is the amount in milk toothpaste. The child would only need a small, pea-sized blob of toothpaste on the toothbrush.

5 For a high-risk child, 1000 ppm would be needed, but the parent must brush the child's teeth twice a day. Topical fluoride application in the form of Duraphat® (2.26%) biannually would also be recommended.

6 Explain that fluoride has been shown to reduce caries experience (tooth decay) by 50%.

7 Fluoride can work on those teeth already erupted in the mouth, but will also have a beneficial effect on developing teeth (ie beneficial for the adult teeth).

8 There is an optimum level of fluoride ingestion. Exceeding this level can lead to problems of fluorosis, ranging from white opacities on the teeth to more severe discolouration and actual pitting of the teeth. Higher levels of fluoride ingestion can lead to toxicity and even death, so people must not exceed the advised dose. It is therefore important

to know the level of fluoride in the drinking water supply before any fluoride supplements are prescribed.

9   The popular press has caused people to think that fluoride will cause cancer – there is no documented evidence to support this claim.

10 The child must spit out after brushing.

11 Rinsing with water after brushing will remove some of the fluoride.

12 Fluoride rinses are not suitable for this age group, as children often swallow the liquid.

Comment

Recommended maximum fluoride dosage (where water contains less than 0.3 ppm fluoride).

Age	Fluoride (mg/day)
6 months to 3 years	0.25
3–6 years	0.50
6 years +	1.00

Table 2.2

CHAPTER 2 Answers

OSCE Station 2.3

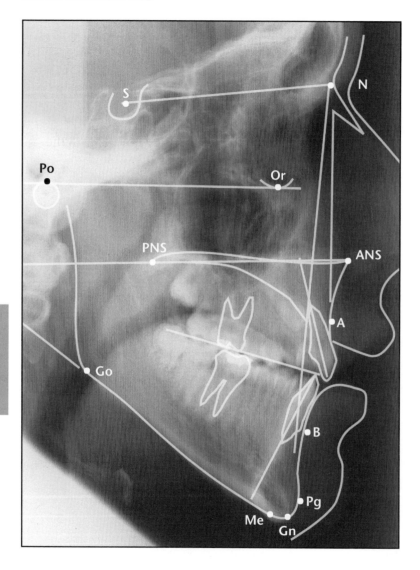

Cephalometric points

S (Sella)	Mid-point of the sella turcica
N (Nasion)	Most anterior point on the fronto-nasal suture
A	Position of maximum concavity on the anterior aspect of the maxilla
B	Position of maximum concavity on the anterior aspect of the mandible
Or (Orbitale)	Most inferior anterior point on orbital rim
Po (Porion)	Uppermost outermost point on bony external auditory meatus
ANS	Anterior nasal spine
PNS	Posterior nasal spine
Go (Gonion)	Most inferior point on the angle of the mandible
Me (Menton)	Lowermost point on the mandibular symphysis
Pg (Pogonion)	Most anterior point on the mandibular symphysis
Gn (Gnathion)	Most anterior and inferior point on the mandibular symphysis
Po–Or	Frankfort plane
PNS–ANS	Maxillary plane
Go–Me	Mandibular plane

OSCE Station 2.4

SNA	82° (± 3)
SNB	79° (± 3)
ANB	3° (± 1)
Upper incisors to maxillary plane	108° (± 5)
Lower incisors to mandibular plane	92° (± 5)
Interincisal angle	133° (± 10)
Maxillomandibular plane angle	27° (± 5)
Lower anterior face height as a percentage of total face height	50–55%

Table 2.4b

The ANB angle is in the range 2–4° in Class I relationships.

The ANB angle is greater than 4° in Class II relationships.

The ANB angle is less than 2° in Class III relationships.

OSCE Station 2.5

1   Introduce yourself politely to the patient and mother.

2   Explain to the patient and mother that the tooth is present and unerupted – this can be done by showing them the radiograph. The tooth is actually palatally placed as shown by the vertical parallax technique. The canine moves in the same direction as the X-ray beam and so is further from the beam than the other teeth in the arch.

3   Explain the possible treatment options:

(i)   Leave alone, but the possible early loss of the primary tooth may leave a space which will need to be filled by a partial denture, bridge or implant when growth has ceased. If the canine is left where it is it will need monitoring to identify any cystic changes associated with the impacted tooth, plus any resorption of adjacent teeth.

(ii) Surgically remove the permanent canine and leave the primary tooth in situ. There is the possibility of damage to adjacent teeth at operation, plus all the common complications of surgical procedures. The patient may not have had experience of dental procedures and so the anaesthetic options will have to be explained.

(iii) Transplant the impacted tooth into the socket of the retained deciduous canine. This is only possible if there is adequate space to fit the larger permanent tooth in the space of the smaller deciduous tooth. The transplant may not be successful, and ankylosis and resorption of the root may occur.

(iv) Orthodontically reposition the tooth. This can be done by either exposing and bonding the tooth or by exposing the tooth followed by pack placement. As the tooth is palatally placed, the option of apically repositioning the flap to expose the tooth is not possible. The patient will need to wear fixed orthodontic appliances to assist the eruption of the tooth. The surgical procedure could be done under local anaesthetic or general anaesthetic, depending on the cooperation of the child. This option would provide the best long-term solution.

4   Ask the patient and mother if they have any questions.

CHAPTER 2
Answers

OSCE Station 2.6

A   Causes of unerupted or missing upper central incisors:

- Extracted or avulsed
- Ectopic position of tooth germ
- Crowding
- Supernumerary
- Dilacerated root
- Pathology (eg cyst, odontome)
- Congenitally absent

B   A midline supernumerary tooth could present by causing:

- Displacement of permanent teeth
- Crowding of permanent teeth
- Midline discrepancies
- Midline diastema
- Root resorption of adjacent teeth

C   Explain the treatment:

1   Introduce yourself politely to the patient.

2   Explain treatment options:

(i)   No treatment – this is not suitable as it has already delayed the eruption of the central incisor.

(ii)   Await eruption of the supernumerary and then extract it – this is not really suitable as the child is now aged 9 and the central incisor has not erupted, and it is unlikely that the supernumerary will erupt of its own accord.

(iii)   Surgical removal of supernumerary and allow the central incisor to erupt. There may not be adequate space for the incisor, in which case orthodontic treatment may be required. Removal will probably need to be done under general anaesthetic as it is still unerupted and the child is aged 9 years. It is necessary to ensure that space is maintained in this region to allow the permanent tooth to erupt. If inadequate space is present, orthodontic treatment to create space may be needed.

(iv) Surgical removal of the supernumerary and bonding of the incisor tooth with a bracket and gold chain to pull it into place. This would probably need to be done under general anaesthesia (GA).

(v) Ask if they have any questions.

OSCE Station 2.7

A

1 Introduce yourself politely to the patient and mother.

2 Establish the nature of accident – how, when and where it occurred.

3 Check that there are no other injuries other than to the tooth. Especially ask about loss of consciousness, nausea, vomiting or dizziness as these may imply a head injury.

4 Establish any past medical/dental history.

5 Check the patient is up to date with vaccinations, in particular tetanus.

6 Warn the parent of possible sequelae:

   (a) To the adjacent primary teeth:

(i) Discolouration – if the teeth become grey early on, the pulp may be vital and the discolouration reversible, but later on may indicate pulp necrosis. Yellow discolouration of the tooth is suggestive of pulp calcification and requires no treatment.

(ii) Pulp death – will require extraction.

   (b) To the permanent teeth (trauma to the primary tooth in 60% of children under 4 years affects their underlying developing permanent tooth, the effect depending on the stage of development, type and severity of injury, treatment and pulpal status): hypomineralisation, hypoplasia, dilacerations, malformations, arrest of development.

7 Invite questions and answer any concerns the parent may have.

B If the child was 10 years old, the avulsed incisor would be a permanent tooth so re-implantation would be indicated:

1 Check the tooth is intact and not fractured.

2 Avoid handling the root surface, remove any contaminant by

gently agitating in saline.

3   Anaesthetise the area with local anaesthetic.

4   Place the tooth in the socket.

5   Compress the buccal and palatal alveolar plate.

6   Splint the re-implanted tooth to adjacent teeth using wire and composite, extending from the upper right central incisor to the upper left lateral incisor.

7   Prescribe antibiotics and chlorhexidine mouthwash.

The patient needs to be reviewed between 7 and 10 days afterwards, when the splinting needs to be removed. Prolonged splinting promotes ankylosis.

Comment

Around 8% of 5-year-olds experience dental trauma, mainly as a toddler. Luxation and displacement injuries are more common in deciduous teeth than root fractures because the alveolar bone is more elastic.

CHAPTER 2
Answers

OSCE Station 2.8

1   Introduce yourself politely to the patient and parent.

2   Establish the circumstances surrounding the injury.

3   Ask if there was any loss of consciousness.

4   Check the patient's medical history including tetanus status.

5   Examine the patient: determine which teeth are mobile; exclude any alveolar fractures.

6   Say to the examiner that another radiograph should be taken at a different angle in order to visualise the fracture.

7   Treatment depends on the position of the fracture:

Position of root fracture	Treatment
Apical 1/3	No treatment unless mobile and displaced coronal fragment If required, reposition and splint for 3–6 weeks Keep under observation for necrosis of coronal pulp to level of root fracture RCT to coronal pulp if non-vital
Middle 1/3	Coronal fragment is usually loose and requires repositioning and splinting for 3–6 weeks If becomes non-vital, RCT to fracture line If requires extraction, leave apical fragment in situ
Coronal 1/3	If possible treat as for middle third root fracture If not, then either extraction of both parts or removal of coronal part and RCT to apical fragment Restoration to prevent gingival overgrowth Permanent restoration: post crown Consider orthodontic extrusion/ gingivectomy if necessary, or overdenture (upper partial denture) and retain root to maintain alveolar bone height

Table 2.8

OSCE Station 2.9

1   Introduce yourself politely to the patient and parent.

2   Take a detailed history, including the patient's complaint and the history of that complaint. As the patient has suffered trauma you will need to check if there were any other injuries or loss of consciousness, vomiting or dizziness.

3   Take a medical history including tetanus status.

4   Carry out a detailed examination, extra-oral and intra-oral, hard and soft tissue.

5   Special tests – radiographs to rule out root or dentoalveolar fractures.

6   Explain that the treatment will depend on the type of fracture, and management will depend on patient tolerance:

- Enamel fracture only: smooth off the sharp edge.
- Enamel and dentine fracture: need to protect the exposed dentine. Use calcium hydroxide lining and an acid-etch retained composite restoration.
- Enamel, dentine and pulp:
  - If there is a tiny exposure, then attempt a direct pulp cap with calcium hydroxide and cover with an acid-etch retained composite restoration.
  - If there is a large exposure, then the tooth will need some form of pulp treatment: (i) Cvek pulpotomy/ partial pulpotomy to try to maintain vitality of the pulp tissue, (ii) coronal pulpectomy or (iii) total pulpectomy as the last option.

Comment

A Cvek pulpotomy is done by removing the exposed and contaminated pulp with a high-speed handpiece with diamond bur and water coolant; calcium hydroxide is placed at the base of the cavity after achieving haemostasis. Glass ionomer cement (GIC) is placed in the remainder of the cavity, then an acid-etch bond and composite restoration is carried out. Follow up at 1, 3 and 6 months. This has a success rate of about 96%.

OSCE Station 2.10

1   Prepare instruments and materials.

2   Anaesthetise the tooth.

3   Isolate the tooth with rubber dam.

4   Prepare the cavity (in order to gain the best access it is important to extend the occlusal part of the cavity to cover the whole of the roof of the pulp chamber).

5   Excavate deep caries.

6   Remove the roof of the pulp chamber with a sterile diamond fissure bur in a high-speed handpiece, taking care to remove overhanging dentine ledges.

7   Remove the coronal pulp with a large excavator or a rose-head bur (size 6/8) in a slow-speed handpiece.

8   Irrigate the pulp chamber with sterile saline or water.

9   Dry and control bleeding with cotton wool.

10 If formocresol is to be used, then dip a pledget of cotton wool in it and remove the excess liquid by dabbing with gauze. Alternatively, use ferric sulphate (15.5%).

11 Place the pledget of formocresol in the pulp chamber over the stumps of the radicular pulp and leave in place for 4–5 minutes. Care must be taken not to allow the formocresol to get onto any soft tissues other than the pulp. If using ferric sulphate, place for 30 seconds.

12 Remove the pledget and place an antiseptic dressing over the remaining pulp stumps. The dressing can be made from zinc oxide and eugenol, by adding an equal amount of formocresol to the eugenol and mixing it with the zinc oxide.

13 Place a cement base over the paste and then restore the tooth. It will need a stainless-steel crown.

14 You can take a check radiograph to ensure that the pulp chamber has been adequately filled.

OSCE Station 2.11

The cause is frequent ingestion of sugar and/or reduced salivary flow. The distribution suggests frequent consumption of sugary drinks from a feeding bottle, or prolonged on-demand breast-feeding.

1   Introduce yourself politely to the patient and establish rapport with the child.

2   Take a detailed history; establish when the decay started.

3   Take any past medical history and establish whether the child is on any sugar-based medication.

4   Confirm the likely cause and obtain a history of sugar intake. A diet sheet is helpful. (See Answer 2.1.)

5   Provide education regarding sugar intake. Suggest that the child should be given only water at night.

6   Discuss fluoride supplementation, either as a paste with 1000 ppm instead of the normal lower dose in children's pastes, or as fluoride supplements.

7   Consider extraction of poor-prognosis primary teeth and painful teeth.

8   Consider restoring teeth that are savable – stainless-steel crowns.

9   Concentrate on prevention in permanent dentition.

10 Encourage the mother to bring her son regularly for further check-ups.

Comment

Rampant caries is sudden-onset and rapidly progressive caries, where many/all teeth are affected and the surfaces involved are not normally affected by caries. Bottle caries characteristically starts with maxillary incisors; the primary molars may be affected in severe cases; the lower incisors are usually spared.

OSCE Station 2.12

1   The wire needs to be bent to fit closely to the labial aspect of the upper anterior teeth.

2   It must fit passively around the upper anterior teeth.

3   It must be extended to at least one tooth on either side of the avulsed incisor, but can be extended further for added stability.

4   In a patient, the wire splint would be held in place with an adhesive material such as acid-etch composite. As the wire is being placed on a stone model, wax can be used instead to mimic the role of the adhesive material.

5   The wax (adhesive material) must be placed so that the ends of the wire are embedded in it to prevent them being sharp.

6   The wax (adhesive material) is placed on the labial aspect of the anterior teeth, usually in the centre of the labial face of the crown.

CHAPTER 2
Answers

OSCE Station 2.13

1   Introduce yourself politely to the mother. You need to remember that the mother is probably upset by the whole episode.

2   Ask how the daughter is now; there may be another injury that is more serious than an avulsed tooth requiring urgent treatment.

3   Ask about the daughter's medical history to check that she is fit and healthy with no contraindications to re-implanting the tooth.

4   Ask what time the accident happened – the sooner the tooth is re-implanted the better.

5   Ask whether the tooth is complete or is in pieces – a fractured tooth is not suitable for re-implantation.

6   The sooner the tooth is replaced the better, so advise the mother to hold the tooth by the crown and gently wash off any debris, such as road grit. This can be done by swishing it in a cup of milk. Do not wipe the root as this will remove periodontal ligament cells.

7   Place the tooth back in the socket with the smooth convex surface facing out of the mouth. If it doesn't seat fully, get the daughter to gently bite on a handkerchief to apply pressure to the area, and come up to the dental practice for splinting of the tooth. If the mother cannot or does not want to replace the tooth, then the tooth needs to be stored in an appropriate solution until re-implantation. Saliva is better than milk, which is better than air. The tooth could be stored by the child placing it in the lower buccal sulcus, BUT they must be careful not to swallow it. The next best thing is to put the tooth in a container of milk and come to the surgery where the tooth can be replaced and splinted.

OSCE Station 2.14

1   Introduce yourself politely to the patient and parent.

2   Establish rapport with child.

- Points to cover include:
- Only used for permanent teeth.
- Fluoride will help reduce caries on smooth surfaces but has little effect on pit and fissure caries; covering these stagnation points with a sealant can prevent caries developing.
- The cost of these sealants is high, so they are only used on high-risk sites.
- Proportion of occlusal decay prevented is about 70% with auto-polymerised sealant.
- About 60% of surfaces treated remain covered after 5–6 years.
- Sealants need to be checked after placement as the probability of loss of the sealant is highest soon after placement.
- The greatest risk of caries in molars appears to be 2–4 years after eruption, but the pits and fissures remain susceptible to caries into adolescence and beyond.
- Teeth should be sealed as soon as possible after eruption, although the tooth will need to be sufficiently erupted to allow rubber dam to be placed.

OSCE Station 2.15

A

1   Show James how to insert and remove the appliance.

2   He should wear the appliance full time for maximum effect, which includes meals and in bed at night.

3   However, if he plays contact sports it may be better to remove it and keep it in a small rigid container.

4   The appliance needs to be cleaned daily, and not just by rinsing it under the tap, but also by brushing it as well. James should not use very hot water or bleach to clean it.

5   James' speech will be altered at first but this should settle down within about 48 hours.

6   For the first couple of days, the brace may feel tight and uncomfortable but this should settle down as well. If needed, James could take analgesics, such as paracetamol or ibuprofen.

7   It is best to avoid sticky and chewy foods such as chewing gum.

8   If the brace breaks or there are problems, James should contact the practice.

B

1   First check how James has got on since the last visit and find out if he has had any problems with his appliance.

2   Check the appliance in the mouth:

- Does it go in and out easily or is it tight? You can also get the patient to remove it, which will give you an idea of proficient he is at handling it.
- Are the active components (springs) still active? This will give you a clue as to whether James has been wearing it as prescribed.

3   Assess any tooth movement since last visit.

CHAPTER 2
Answers

4   Check the appliance for damage.

5   To adjust the appliance:

- Activate the active components by bending the wire spring. You are aiming for 1 mm tooth movement per month. With a palatal finger spring of 0.5 mm wire this will be about 3–4 mm of movement on the spring. If in doubt you can measure the force with a gauge – you are aiming for 30–40 g.
- Check the retention of the appliance and adjusts the cribs as necessary.
- Adjust the baseplate if necessary.

6   Check the appliance in the mouth for active components and retention.

7   Repeat instructions on care and reinforce oral hygiene instructions.

C

Points to note are:

- Check if his speech is altered, he may lisp or slur his words as he is not used to wearing the appliance.
- There is little or no movement of teeth since the last appointment and the springs are still active.
- The appliance looks new.
- James is not proficient at inserting the appliance.
- The appliance is not a good fit.
- There is no imprint of the arrowheads of the Adams' cribs on the gingivae.
- There is no outline of the baseplate on the palatal mucosa.

OSCE Station 2.16

A

The patient has missing upper lateral incisors and a crossbite on the left side.

B

Causes of missing incisors:

- Developmentally absent
- Previously extracted
- Avulsed (unlikely as bilateral)
- Dilacerated/displaced due to trauma (unlikely as bilateral)
- Supernumerary teeth preventing eruption
- Crowding – insufficient space
- Pathological lesion.

C

Management would be as follows:

1 Introduce yourself politely to the patient.

2 From the history determine whether the teeth were ever present or have been removed.

3 Ask about any history of trauma.

4 Ask about any family history of missing teeth

5 Check the patient's medical history

6 Do a thorough intra-oral examination; (look for possible unerupted teeth (bulge of unerupted tooth), check the centre line and any crossbite).

7 Assess for periodontal health and look for evidence of caries.

8 Special investigations: Take radiographs (DPT, long-cone periapical radiographs or standard upper occlusal views).

9 A diagnosis can now be made.

10 Discuss the treatment options with the patient, answering any questions that they may have.

11 Take informed consent.

12 Treatment – The various options for treatment depend on the cause and it is important to determine what the patient's wishes are. The treatment options are:

- Leave the problem alone (do nothing).
- Unerupted tooth:
  - Leave as is
  - Orthodontic repositioning – simple exposure or exposure and bonding
  - Transplantation
- Dilacerated tooth – extract and treat as missing tooth.
- Missing tooth/replacement of missing teeth:
  - Partial denture
  - Adhesive bridge
  - Single tooth implant
- Orthodontics to align the canines and camouflage – unlikely to be successful as the patient does not have crowding.

OSCE Station 2.17

The referral letter should be addressed to Consultant Orthodontist. It must include:

- Your contact details, ie address and telephone number
- The patient's details, ie name, date of birth, address and telephone number
- A brief synopsis of the concerns/problem, patient's wishes and a provisional diagnosis. A sample letter is shown below.

Dr A.N. Other,
Smiles Dental Practice,
21 Borough End Road,
Thamestown,
AB1 2CD
Telephone 020 7123 4567

Mr Wire,
Orthodontic Department,
Thamestown General Hospital,
High Street,
Thamestown,
AB3 4CD

Re: Freddy Smith, DOB 13/8/1994, 54 Burntash Avenue, Thamestown AB18 4CD. Telephone 020 7123 9876

Dear Mr Wire,

I would be most grateful if you could see Freddy.
He presented to the practice for routine dental review.
He is complaining of occasional soreness in his palate and his mother is concerned about the appearance of his teeth. Freddy is medically fit and healthy.

Examination reveals a Class II division 1 incisor malocclusion, complicated by an increased overjet (8 mm) and a deep and complete traumatic overbite. He has an IOTN Grade 4 Dental Health Component. His oral hygiene is good with no active decay.

I would appreciate your opinion on the management of his malocclusion.

Yours sincerely,

Dr A.N. Other

Note: The IOTN has two components – the Dental Health Component and the Aesthetic Component. The IOTN must be used now to assess the need and eligibility of children under 18 years of age for NHS orthodontic treatment on dental health grounds.

The Dental Health Component has five grades and looks at traits that may affect the function and longevity of the dentition: from grade 1 (no need) to grade 5 (very great need).

Grades 1–2: little or no treatment need
Grade 3: possible need for treatment
Grades 4-5: definite need for treatment

The Aesthetic Component attempts to assess the aesthetic handicap of the malocclusion and consists of a scale of 10 colour photographs of teeth showing different levels of dental attractiveness. The grading is done by the orthodontist by matching the patient's teeth with the photographs. In the NHS, the Aesthetic Component is used to determine need for treatment for border-line cases with grade 3 DHC. If the case has a high Aesthetic Component score, NHS treatment is permissible.

With regards to treatment needs the Aesthetic Component scores are:

Score 1–2: no treatment
Score 3–4: slight
Score 5–6: moderate/borderline
Score 8–10: definite

CHAPTER 2
Questions

CHAPTER 2
Answers

PERIODONTOLOGY

Chapter 3: Questions

OSCE Station 3.1
5 minute station

This 50-year-old man attends your practice complaining of painful gums, along with a metallic taste. On examination he has poor oral hygiene with yellowish-white ulcers, in particular in the interdental papillae.

How would you manage this patient? What is the likely diagnosis?

OSCE Station 3.2
5 minute station

Please give oral hygiene advice to this adult patient.

OSCE Station 3.3
5 minute station

This patient presents with pain in the lower right second premolar. Radiographs show a periapical radiolucency and loss of bone height.

How would you determine whether this is a periodontal or a periapical lesion?

OSCE Station 3.4
5 minute station

A patient presents with grade 1 mobility of the lower right first permanent molar. There is clinical evidence of furcation involvement.

A   How would you classify furcation involvement?

B   What treatment is available for this condition?

OSCE Station 3.5
5 minute station

An 18-year-old woman presents with a missing central incisor following trauma. She currently wears an acrylic partial denture and wishes to know what treatment options are available to replace her missing tooth. Please explain the treatment options to the patient.

OSCE Station 3.6
5 minute station

A 14-year-old girl attends your practice as a new patient. On examination she has reasonable oral hygiene, but there are pockets around her central incisors and first molars, with drifting of the incisors.

A   What disease could she have and how would you manage it?

B   What possible complications are associated with the medical management of this condition?

OSCE Station 3.7
5 minute station

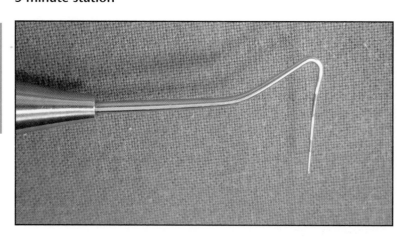

A What type of probe is shown here?

B At what level does the coloured band on the probe lie?

C You have carried out a periodontal examination of a patient in your dental surgery. The worst results per sextant are as follows:

- Upper right first molar – pocket (2 mm only)
- Upper central incisor – pocket (2mm only)
- Upper left first molar – pocket (2 mm) with a subgingival overhang
- Lower right first molar – pocket (5 mm)
- Lower central incisor – gingival bleeding but no pockets
- Lower left first molar – pocket (6 mm)

Please score the results according to the BPE (Basic Periodontal Examination).

0	0	2
3	1	4

Table 3.7a

D What treatment would be appropriate for this patient?

OSCE Station 3.8
5 minute station

This 24-year-old woman presents at your practice complaining of bleeding gums. The history reveals that she is in the second trimester of pregnancy, and that otherwise she is fit and healthy.

A How would you manage her problem?

B What other problems may she have/develop and how are they managed?

CHAPTER 3
Questions

OSCE Station 3.9
5 minute station

A patient attends your practice and requires extensive scaling. She has previously only experienced hand scaling and wishes to know why you are planning on using an ultrasonic scaler. Please explain the advantages and disadvantages of hand versus ultrasonic scaling to her.

OSCE Station 3.10
5 minute station

A 50-year-old man presents to your practice with a bridge extending from the upper right first premolar to the upper left first premolar. The abutment teeth are mobile, as are the remaining molar teeth. The patient has a strong gag reflex and has non-insulin-dependent diabetes. He wishes to know whether he could have dental implants and what factors influence the success/failure of dental implants. Please discuss with him the pros and cons of replacing his tooth-retained bridge with an implant-retained bridge.

Chapter 3: Answers

OSCE Station 3.1

1 Introduce yourself politely to the patient.

2 Obtain a brief history of the complaint.

3 Determine if there are any associated risk factors.

4 Explain to the examiner that you would usually examine the patient. The likely diagnosis is necrotising ulcerative gingivitis and so further management would include an explanation to the patient etc.

5 Explain to the patient that it is important to achieve good plaque control. Discuss the following:

   (a) Oral hygiene instructions (although the patient may not be able to brush teeth adequately due to pain).

   (b) If possible, carry out full-mouth supragingival ultrasonic instrumentation for reducing plaque mass; if it is not possible due to pain it could be done a week later.

   (c) Chemical plaque control – chlorhexidine mouthwash.

   (d) Metronidazole 200–400 mg three times daily for 3 days.

   (e) Once acute symptoms have resolved, then further full-mouth root surface instrumentation to remove all of the deposits on the teeth and reiterate oral hygiene instructions.

6 Give advice regarding management of risk factors – oral hygiene, smoking cessation and stress management.

7 Consider referral to a specialist centre.

Comment

Necrotising ulcerative gingivitis is extremely painful and associated with spirochaetal infection, smoking and stress, and possibly human immunodeficiency virus (HIV) infection.

CHAPTER 3
Answers

OSCE Station 3.2

Adults may be embarrassed by receiving instructions on oral hygiene, so the method of delivery is important.

1   Introduce yourself politely to the patient.

2   Explain that brushing is important for the prevention and control of tooth decay and gum disease.

3   Advise that they should aim to brush twice daily with fluoride toothpaste. Different fluoride preparations have similar efficacy.

4   Explain that they should try to limit rinsing with water after brushing as this washes the fluoride away.

5   Explain that they should try to brush last thing at night before going to bed.

6   For patients with periodontal disease, brushing with tooth-pastes containing triclosan with either copolymer or zinc cit-rate results in improved levels of plaque control and periodontal health.

7   Studies on the different toothbrushing techniques have yielded different results. It may be better to try to improve the technique that the patient already uses rather than to introduce a new one, provided that it is not likely to be damaging to the oral tissues.

8   Information on different brushing and hygiene aids is also useful.

   •   Toothbrushes should have a small head with soft, rounded bristles. If the patient does not have the manual dexterity to use a manual toothbrush, then an electric toothbrush can be used. However, a normal healthy adult patient should have adequate manual dexterity to use a manual toothbrush.
   •   Standard toothbrushes do not reach the interdental regions and so an alternative device is needed for these areas.
   •   Flossing is the best method when the papilla fills the inter-dental space. However, it does require manual dexterity

and is time-consuming. For patients with open interdental spaces an interdental bottlebrush is ideal.
- A single-tuft interspace brush is good for cleaning around tipped or rotated teeth or teeth adjacent to an extraction site. It is of limited value for cleaning between teeth that are in normal alignment.
- Toothpicks (wood points), like interspace brushes, are only effective when there is space between the teeth.

9   Chemical plaque removal with mouthwashes:

- Chlorhexidine works by preventing development of supragingival plaque. It does not affect established gingivitis where subgingival plaque is present. It also has some side-effects such as altered taste and staining of teeth, so is not recommended for long-term use except in special circumstances.
- Pre-brushing rinses are available, but their value is debatable.

Comment

The adult dental health survey of 1998 showed that the prevalence of plaque and periodontal disease in the UK remains high: 72% of dentate adults and 33% of teeth had visible plaque and 54% of adults had pocket depth greater than 3.5 mm. If large numbers of teeth are to be retained into old age there is a need to improve the oral cleanliness of the majority of the population in the UK.

CHAPTER 3
Answers

OSCE Station 3.3

1 Introduce yourself politely to the patient.

2 Take a pain history and establish the nature of the pain.

3 Examine the patient and assess response to percussion and vitality testing.

4 Assess pocket depth.

Comment

- Periodontal and periapical pathologies can occur together which may lead to difficulty in diagnosis. There is little evidence to support the theory that periodontal pathology leads to pulpal necrosis.
- As in most clinical situations, to reach a diagnosis the clinician must take an appropriate history, followed by examination and investigation, starting with chair-side investigations (eg vitality testing) followed by special investigations (radiological).

	Primarily periodontal	Primarily pulpal
History	No preceding toothache	Often have toothache
Percussion	Tooth tender on percussion, especially laterally	Tooth tender on percussion vertically
Probing	Periodontal pockets present	No pockets
Probing sinus	May lead to pocket	May lead to apex
Discharge	Through pocket	Usually over apex; may be at gingival margin
Swelling	In attached gingiva	At apex
Timing	Swelling usually precedes pain	Pain usually precedes swelling
Vitality testing	Usually positive	Negative
Radiographs	Vertical bone loss	Apical area

Table 3.3

OSCE Station 3.4

A Furcation involvement occurs where periodontal disease extends into the bifurcation or trifurcation area of multi-rooted teeth.

	Classification of		
	First degree	**Second degree**	**Third degree**
	Horizontal loss of bone support not exceeding 1/3 of the tooth width	Horizontal loss of bone support > 1/3 of the tooth width but not total width of furcation area	Horizontal through-and-through destruction in furcation area
Treatment	Scaling and root planning ± furcationplasty	Furcationplasty ± tunnel preparation ± root resection or extraction	Tunnel preparation ± root resection or extraction

Table 3.4

B Treatments available for furcation involvement include:

- Scaling and root debridement – This is successful only if the patient is able to keep the area clean post-treatment.
- Furcationplasty – This is a surgical procedure involving a mucoperiosteal flap that allows root planning and scaling followed by removal of tooth structure in the furcation area. This enables access for cleaning. Recontouring of the bone may be required. There is a risk of sensitivity and caries.
- Tunnel preparation – Buccal and lingual flaps are raised, the entire furcation area is exposed and the flaps are approximated with inter-radicular sutures, leaving a large exposed furcation. There is a risk of sensitivity, caries and pulpal exposure.
- Root resection – This involves the amputation of one or more roots of a multi-rooted tooth, leaving the crown and root stump. The root to be retained needs endodontic treatment.

CHAPTER 3
Answers

- Hemisection – This involves sectioning of a two-rooted tooth to give two smaller units, each with a single root. Root canal treatment is necessary pre-operatively and restoration of the crown post-operatively.
- Guided tissue regeneration – This involves interposition of a barrier to epithelial migration prior to completion of surgical or non-surgical treatment to encourage new connective tissue attachment. The effectiveness of this technique is under review.
- Enamel matrix derivatives – These substances may help formation of acellular cementum and are locally applied to the root surface. However, they are more commonly used on single-rooted teeth.

OSCE Station 3.5

1   Introduce yourself politely to the patient.

2   Find out what she is concerned about. Is the appearance a problem, or the smile line, or does she want a non-removable option?

3   Check the patient's medical history eg conditions such as diabetes and whether she is a smoker as this may influence the ultimate decision.

4   Explain to the examiner that you would then proceed to examine the patient.

5   Discuss the following options:

- Resin-bonded bridge
- Conventional bridge
- Single-tooth implant

Resin bridge

Advantages:
- Minimal tooth preparation
- No need for local anaesthetic
- Cheaper than conventional bridge
- Fixed prosthesis

Disadvantages:
- Can debond
- Metal may show through the abutments

Conventional bridge

Advantages:
- Good aesthetics
- Better retention compared with resin bridge
- Fixed prosthesis

Disadvantages:
- More tooth preparation compared with adhesive bridge
- Often involves a full-coverage crown on the abutment tooth
- Risk of pulpal damage

Single-tooth implant

Advantages:
- Fixed prosthesis
- Good aesthetics and functional outcome
- No preparation of adjacent teeth
- Good success rates reported

Disadvantages:
- Expensive
- Staged procedure, time-consuming
- Needs temporary replacement during osseo-integration
- May require bone augmentation, depending on alveolar bone volume

OSCE Station 3.6

A The patient has localised aggressive periodontitis. Management of LJP includes:

- Meticulous oral hygiene
- Scaling and root planing ± access flap surgery
- Consider antibiotics – systemic or local
  - Doxycycline 100 mg once daily for 2–3 weeks
  - Oxytetracycline 250 mg four times daily for 2–3 weeks
  - 400 mg metronidazole three times a day
  - Locally deposited slow-release tetracycline (Dentomycin gel)

B Tetracyclines deposit in developing teeth causing staining and hypoplasia, so should be avoided in children under 12 years and in pregnancy.

Comment

- Once the disease is stabilised, orthodontics can be considered if any teeth have drifted.
- LJP occurs in childhood and adolescence and is usually localised to the incisors and first molars. The gingivae may look normal despite the presence of deep periodontal pockets. The degree of periodontal destruction is out of proportion to the deposits of plaque and calculus. Many organisms have been implicated: mainly *Actinobacillus actinomycetem comitans* (Aa); others include *Eubacterium* and *Bacteroides*-like species. LJP is more common in girls, Afro-Caribbeans, and is often familial. Prevalence is low, approximately 0.2%.
- Tetracyclines are active against Aa and many other periodontal pathogens. Their actions include reduction of host neutrophil collagenase and reduction of bone loss, in addition to the antibacterial action. High concentrations are found in crevicular fluid.

OSCE Station 3.7

A The World Health Organization (WHO) periodontal probe – ball-ended, with a diameter of 0.5 mm.

B The coloured band lies 3.5–5.5 mm from the tip.

C The scoring system is as follows:

Score	Disease	Treatment
0	No disease	
1	No pockets > 3 mm, no overhangs or calculus but gingival bleeding occurs after probing	Oral hygiene instruction (OHI)
2	No pockets > 3 mm; subgingival calculus present or subgingival overhangs	OHI, scaling and correction of any iatrogenic factors
3	Deepest pocket > 3.5 mm but < 5.5 mm	OHI, scaling and root planning
4	One or more tooth in the sextant has a pocket > 6 mm	OHI, scaling and root planning ± surgery as required
NB	Furcation or total loss of attachment of 7 mm or more	Need to carry out a full periodontal examination regardless of CPITN* score

Table 3.7b
*CPITN, Community Periodontal Index of Treatment Needs.

This patient would score:

0	0	2
3	1	4

Table 3.7c

D The treatment needed is shown in the table below:

		OHI, scaling and treatment of any iatrogenic problems
OHI, scaling and root planning	OHI	OHI, scaling, root planning ± surgery

Table 3.7d

OSCE Station 3.8

1 Introduce yourself politely to the patient.

2 Explain that you will be carrying out a full intra-oral examination to determine plaque levels, along with evaluation of gingival and periodontal health.

3 Explain that gingival inflammation initiated by plaque is exacerbated by hormonal changes in pregnancy, especially during the second and third trimesters.

A Management includes:

- Establishment of effective oral hygiene
- Subgingival scaling
- Regular supportive care

B Pregnancy can be associated with various periodontal conditions, including:

- Pyogenic granuloma
- Marked pregnancy gingivitis
- Worsening of existing periodontitis
- Physiological increase in tooth mobility towards the end of pregnancy
- Pregnancy diabetes
- Vitamin deficiency

Comment

A pyogenic granuloma or pregnancy epulis is a pedunculated, fibrogranulomatous lesion that usually occurs in the anterior maxillary interdental papillae. It bleeds easily when traumatised. Management during pregnancy includes careful oral hygiene and debridement. These lesions are best removed after parturition, when there is often considerable reduction in size.

OSCE Station 3.9

1   Introduce yourself politely to the patient.

2   Explain the advantages and disadvantages of hand scaling versus ultrasonic scaling:

Ultrasonic instrumentation	Hand instrumentation
Faster	Slower
Can be uncomfortable	May be more comfortable
Several mechanisms of action: cavitation, acoustic turbulence, fluid lavage and mechanical action	Mechanical action
Ability to disrupt and destroy bacteria from a distance	Can only remove what it touches
Small tip size (0.3–0.6 mm)	Larger tip size (0.76–1.0 mm)
Tip has 360° circle of activity	Only cutting edge is capable of calculus removal
Light lateral and relaxed pressure is used for calculus removal	Moderate–firm lateral pressure is needed for calculus removal
Easily inserted into pockets with minimal stretching of pocket wall	Must be positioned apical to deposit, resulting in distension of pocket wall
Limited tissue trauma and faster healing rate	Tissue trauma and slow healing rate
Limited cementum removal	Cementum removal
Can leave rough root surface	Smoother root surface
No sharpening of instruments required	Frequent sharpening of instruments required

Table 3.9

CHAPTER 3
Answers

OSCE Station 3.10

1 Introduce yourself politely to the patient.

2 Explain the advantages and disadvantages of implants and dentures:

Advantages of implants	Advantages of a denture
Will provide a stable prosthesis	Cost
Can be fixed or removable	No surgery
Can be tolerated by patients with a gag reflex	
Maintains supporting bone	
Disadvantages of implants	**Disadvantages of a denture**
Surgical procedure	Is not a fixed prosthesis
Take longer to produce from start to finish than a denture	Must be removed at night
Cost	May be unstable and unretentive
Maintenance requirements	
Must have adequate bone and so may need a bone graft	May not be tolerated if the patient has a gag reflex
Poorer prognosis in people with diabetes (see below)	Bone will resorb with time
Poor prognosis in smokers	

Table 3.10

Diabetes

Loss of the periodontal attachment occurs more frequently in people with moderate to poorly controlled diabetes (type 1 or type 2) than in those with better control. Diabetic patients with more advanced systemic complications have greater frequency and severity of periodontal disease. Although implants do not have a periodontal ligament they are still subject to peri-implantitis, and as such there is at greater risk in a diabetic patient. The better controlled the diabetes, the better the prognosis.

RESTORATIVE DENTISTRY AND DENTAL MATERIALS

Chapter 4: Questions

OSCE Station 4.1
5 minute station

A Please mix some zinc phosphate cement to use as a base material.

B Why is it mixed on a glass slab?

Props:

- Glass slab
- Zinc phosphate powder and dispenser
- Zinc phosphate liquid
- Mixing spatula

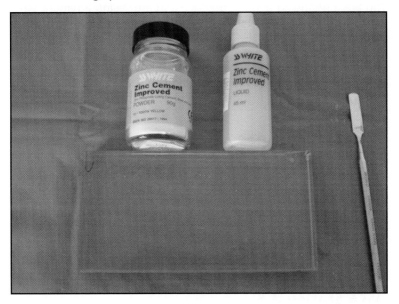

OSCE Station 4.2
5 minute station

Please take a facebow recording for this patient.

Props:

- Facebow with occlusal fork
- Dental wax
- Hot water to soften wax
- Labels

OSCE Station 4.3
5 minute station

You are a dentist in general practice and are seeing a patient who wears a chrome upper partial denture. The patient has denture stomatitis on the palate.

Please explain what the problem is and how you would treat this condition. Please explain the treatment to the patient.

OSCE Station 4.4
5 minute station

A 16-year-old girl attends your surgery concerned about the appearance of her front teeth. She has evidence of loss of tooth substance on the labial and palatal surfaces of her anterior teeth.

How would you manage this patient?

OSCE Station 4.5
5 minute station

You are a dentist in general practice. While carrying out root canal therapy on an upper molar you fracture a file in the canal.

Explain how you would proceed and how you would explain the problem to the patient.

OSCE Station 4.6
5 minute station

You are a dentist in general practice. While carrying out root canal therapy on a molar you cause a traumatic perforation.

Explain how you would proceed and how you would explain the problem to the patient.

OSCE Station 4.7
5 minute station

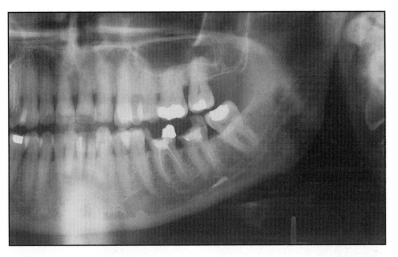

Look at this radiograph.

A   What complication has occurred?

B   What symptoms might the patient be experiencing?

C   What are the other causes of these symptoms?

OSCE Station 4.8
5 minute station

This patient has come to your dental surgery and wants to know about the advantages and disadvantages of composite restorations over amalgam ones.

Please explain the advantages and disadvantages of each material to the patient.

OSCE Station 4.9
5 minute station

Please draw the envelope of motion of the mandible from a point on the tip of a mandibular incisor from a side view (ie in the sagittal plane), and explain the movements.

OSCE Station 4.10
5 minute station

Please mix this glass ionomer cement to use as a luting cement.

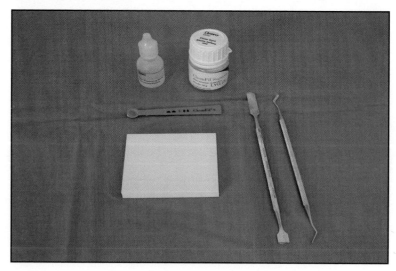

Props:

- Glass ionomer powder/liquid system
- Mixing pad
- Mixing spatula

OSCE Station 4.11
5 minute station

A 24-year-old woman presents to your dental practice with discoloured teeth.

A List four causes of intrinsic tooth discoloration.

B The patient wishes to know what treatment options are available – please discuss them with her.

OSCE Station 4.12
5 minute station

A What types of post and core are available?

B Please give one advantage and disadvantage for each type.

OSCE Station 4.13
5 minute station

A Please do a vitality test of this lower first premolar, explaining what you are doing.

B What could cause a false-negative or false-positive response?

Props:

- Cotton-wool pledget
- Ethyl chloride
- Gutta percha
- Heat source

- Petroleum jelly (Vaseline®)
- Prophylaxis paste
- Electric pulp tester

OSCE Station 4.14
5 minute station

Please isolate this first permanent molar to commence endodontic treatment and explain what you are doing.

Props:

- Phantom head
- Rubber dam sheets
- Assorted clamps
- Dental floss
- Dental wedges
- Gauze squares
- Cotton-wool rolls
- High-speed suction
- Parachute chain

OSCE Station 4.15
5 minute station

A Please survey these study models.

B What is surveying and why is it done?

Props:

- Surveyor with attachments
- Study models

OSCE Station 4.16
5 minute station

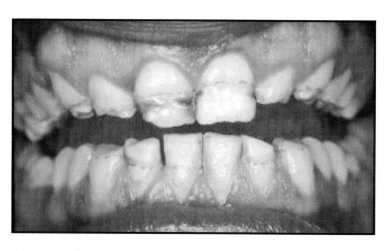

A 35-year-old man presents to your surgery as he is concerned regarding the appearance of his teeth. Please take a history from the patient to ascertain their concerns and to determine the likely cause(s) for the appearance of the teeth.

OSCE Station 4.17
5 minute station

A What is the most likely cause for the appearance of the teeth in the figure in OSCE Station 4.16?

B What treatment may be possible to improve their appearance?

C Please describe the advantages and disadvantages of each briefly to the patient.

OSCE Station 4.18
5 minute station

You are making a full gold crown for a lower left first permanent molar. The crown has come back from the laboratory. Please go through the stages of trying in a crown and cementing it on the dental manikin using the cement provided. Please treat the manikin as though it was a living patient.

Props:

- Dental manikin with crown preparation on lower left first permanent molar tooth
- Full coverage crown on die
- Articulating paper
- Cement
- Dental instruments.

OSCE Station 4.19
5 minute station

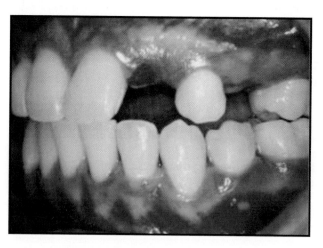

A fit and healthy 35-year-old woman presents to your clinic. She is wearing a partial denture in the place of a missing lateral incisor. She is keen to have a fixed prosthesis. Please discuss her treatment options with her and explain what investigations you need to carry out prior to treatment planning.

Chapter 4: Answers

OSCE Station 4.1

A

1   First the mixing slab shoud be chilled. Dispense the powder and liquid according to the manufacturer's instructions.

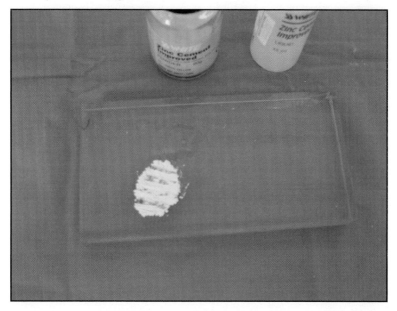

2   The powder should be added to the liquid in increments, mixing for about 10–15 seconds with each increment. It should take about two minutes in total.

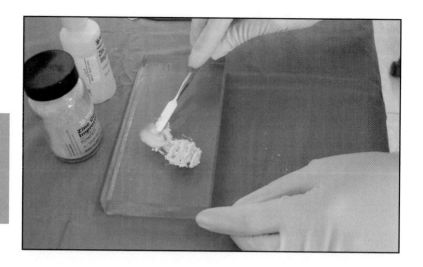

3   A large area of the mixing slab should be used in an effort to dissipate the heat of the exothermic setting reaction.

4   A figure-of-eight mixing movement should be used.

5   The final mixture should be thick enough to be rolled into a ball with fingers covered in cement powder.

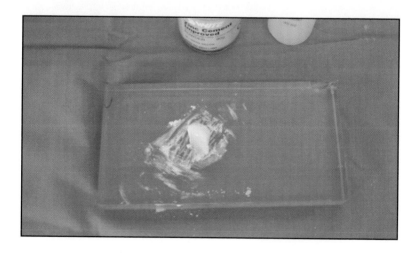

6   The material should be removed from the spatula and slab before it sets as it is very difficult to remove once set.

B   The cement is mixed on a glass slab because of the exothermic setting reaction. The slab can be chilled to absorb the heat and slow the reaction, allowing further increments to be added.

OSCE Station 4.2

1 Introduce yourself politely to the patient and explain what you are going to do, and gain their permission.

2 Check you have all the required equipment.

3 Soften the wax on the occlusal fork in hot water. Check that the wax is not too hot before putting it into the patient's mouth.

4 Position the occlusal fork onto the occlusal surface of the upper teeth with the central marking (if present) in the midline. Allow the wax to cool.

5 Insert the occlusal fork handle into a clamp on the facebow.

6 Adjust the facebow to:

(a) Locate the condyles, 12 mm anterior to the tragus of the ear. Centre the facebow on the face.

(b) Record the relationship of the occlusal plane to the Frankfort plane (warn the patient that you will be passing the orbital pointer towards their eye). Some facebows also record the intercondylar distance.

7 Once the adjustments are complete, tighten the clamp holding the occlusal fork and orbital pointer. Release the condylar rods and remove the facebow from the patient. Check that the clamps are tight.

8 Label the facebow with the patient's name.

Comment

A facebow records the relationship of the upper dental arch to the condylar axis. With the facebow in the top picture the condyle location and centring of the facebow is achieved by adjusting the condylar rods so that the tips contact the skin overlying the condyle and the readings on each rod are equal.

The relation of the occlusal plane to the Frankfort plane is recorded by positioning the orbital pointer so that the tip contacts the skin overlying the lowest point on the intra-orbital margin.

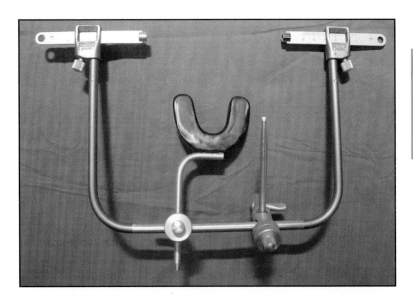

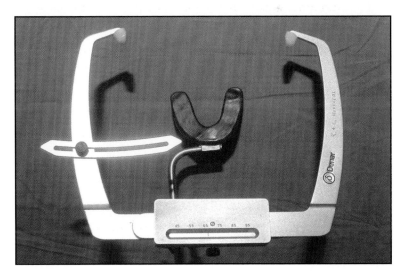

Some facebow designs use the external auditory meatus as a locating structure rather than the condyles and use a point on the face 43 mm above the incisal edge of the upper right central or lateral incisor as the anterior reference point.

OSCE Station 4.3

1   Introduce yourself politely to the patient.

2   *Candida albicans* is a yeast (fungus) that commonly causes infections in the oral cavity.

3   It is present in about 40% of the general population.

4   It can colonise the surface of dentures, especially when dentures are kept in the mouth overnight.

5   This is a common condition, affecting up to 30% of patients wearing full dentures.

6   It is more common in females than males and usually occurs with upper dentures.

7   It does not appear to be transmissible.

8   Explain that their mucosa needs time to recover overnight and so the dentures should be left out – you can liken it to sleeping in your shoes.

9   The dentures must be cleaned thoroughly. This involves cleaning them with a brush and soaking them for at least 15 minutes twice a day in chlorhexidine solution (hypochlorite will discolour the chromework and is used for acrylic dentures).

10 An antifungal cream can be applied to the fitting surface of the denture four times a day.

11 Systemic antifungals should be reserved for patients whose condition does not resolve with topical antifungals.

12 Arrange a review appointment to ensure that these measures are working.

13 Ask the patient if they have any questions.

OSCE Station 4.4

1   Introduce yourself politely to the patient.

2   From the history determine the timescale of tooth substance loss.

3   Determine the cause:

   (a) Dietary – This is likely to cause erosion on the labial surfaces of the incisors first.

   (b) Gastric reflux and bulimia – This causes a pattern of wear on the palatal surfaces of upper incisors, as the gastric acid is thought to strike the palatal surface of the teeth first. However, in severe cases the distinction is less obvious.

   (c) Attrition – This is wear of tooth substance by teeth, which could be caused by bruxism. It usually occurs in conjunction with erosion, but also with abrasion.

   (d) Abrasion – This is wear of the teeth by surfaces other than teeth, for example a toothbrush.

4   Take clinical records, study models and photographs in order to have a baseline record.

5   Discuss prevention of further progression by explanation of the condition and its causes, and the removal of causative factors; referral to a physician for gastrointestinal problems or a psychiatrist for an eating disorder.

6   Monitor if not severe.

7   If severe or if the condition progresses, consider glass ionomer or resin restorations to improve aesthetics or full crowns if wear is excessive.

8   Referral to a restorative specialist if complex restorative problem.

OSCE Station 4.5

1   Calmly explain to the patient that a fine instrument has broken in the canal and that you will try to remove it.

2   If you can see the broken file, try to grasp it with a pair of fine mosquito forceps.

3   Take a radiograph to determine the position.

4   Try to dislodge the broken file by passing a fine file alongside.

5   If this fails, consider trying a Masseran kit.

6   If still not successful, explain to the patient that it is not possible to remove the broken instrument and that you will arrange for a referral to a specialist who will aim to remove the file and/or complete the root canal treatment. The specialist may then attempt to dislodge/remove the broken file with ultrasonic instrumentation. It may be possible for the specialist to create enough space to bypass the fragment by gently working a small file alongside the fractured instrument using EDTA to soften the dentine. If it is not possible to bypass the instrument, then the specialist may clean and fill the root canal to the level of the blockage.

7   Explain that the tooth will need to be kept under observation as it may be necessary to carry out an apicectomy at a later stage.

8   Ask the patient if they have any questions and then arrange a follow-up appointment to see them.

9   Record carefully the event/explanation in the clinical notes.

Comment

Early referral to a specialist may be indicated, depending on the practitioner's experience.

OSCE Station 4.6

1   Calmly ascertain the position and size of the perforation by taking a radiograph.

2   Determine why the perforation occurred. Was access poor? Correct this if possible.

3   Explain to the patient that the above has occurred. Explain that the aim is to seal off the perforation.

4   Discuss the options available and likely outcome and why you think this has happened.

5   Consider early referral to a specialist.

6   Record carefully the event/explanation in the clinical notes.

Treatment options

Pulp chamber perforation

- Small perforation – If bleeding can be arrested, attempt repair using either MTA (mineral tri-oxide aggregate) or glass ionomer cement (GIC). Some suggest using calcium hydroxide but this may wash out.
- Larger perforation – If still restorable, then as above. If not restorable may require hemisection/extraction of tooth.

Lateral perforation

- Gingival third – Incorporate in final restoration, eg diaphragm post and core crown or consider crown lengthening procedure.
- Middle third – Clean and prepare the remainder of the canal by passing instruments down the wall opposite perforation. Fill the canal using a lateral condensation technique and try to occlude the perforation. For larger perforations proceed to fill the root if the bleeding can be arrested. It may require a surgical approach and in multi-rooted teeth hemisection/extraction of the tooth may be necessary.
- Apical third – Clean canal well with sodium hypochlorite

and proceed to fill the root. Consider the vertical condensation technique to attempt to fill both the perforation and the remainder of the canal. If unsuccessful an apicectomy will be required.

Comment

Perforations may be induced by iatrogenic causes, resorptive processes or caries. Lateral perforations often occur as a result of poor access. Apical perforation makes the obturation of the canal difficult.

CHAPTER 4
Answers

OSCE Station 4.7

A   There is radio-opaque matter in the inferior dental canal beneath the lower second molar. This tooth also has some radio-opaque material in the distal root canal. A root canal filling was being carried out and material has extruded through the apex of the tooth and has ended up in the inferior dental canal.

B   If material is in the inferior dental canal it is likely that the patient will complain of altered sensation in the distribution of the inferior dental nerve, ie the lower lip. The altered sensation may be numbness (anaesthesia) or tingling (paraesthesia) and in some cases pain.

C   Other causes of altered sensation:

- Iatrogenic – trauma following surgery, eg surgical removal of wisdom teeth, lower premolars
- Infection – osteomyelitis
- Degenerative – multiple sclerosis
- Metabolic – tetany, diabetic neuropathy
- Neoplastic – space-occupying lesion

OSCE Station 4.8

1 Introduce yourself to the patient.

2 Explain the advantages and disadvantages of composite restorations compared with amalgam restorations.

Advantages of composite restorations

- Aesthetic.
- Conservative removal of tooth structure (less extension; uniform depth not necessary; mechanical retention not usually necessary).
- Less complex when preparing the tooth.
- Provides insulation, has low thermal conductivity.
- Bonds to the tooth structure, resulting in good retention, low microleakage, minimal interfacial staining and increased strength of remaining tooth.
- Repairable.

Disadvantages of composite restorations

- Potential for gap formation as a result of polymerisation shrinkage.
- More difficult, time-consuming and costly compared with amalgam because:
  - treatment usually requires multiple steps;
  - insertion is more difficult (depth of cure is limited);
  - establishing proximal contact, axial contours, embrasures and occlusal contacts may be more difficult; and finishing and polishing procedures are more difficult.
- More technique-sensitive (isolation, etchant, primer and adhesive).
- May exhibit greater occlusal wear in areas of high occlusal stress or when all of the tooth's occlusal contacts are on the composite material.
- Have a higher linear coefficient of thermal expansion, resulting in potential marginal percolation if inadequate bonding technique is ultilised.

Advantages of amalgam restorations

- Ease of use.
- High compressive strength.
- Excellent wear resistance.
- Favourable long-term clinical research result.
- Lower cost than for composite restorations.

Disadvantages of amalgam restorations

- Not aesthetic.
- No insulation.
- Less conservative (more removal of tooth structure during tooth preparation).
- Weakens the tooth structure (unless bonded).
- Initial microleakage.
- More difficult tooth preparation.

Comment

Bonded amalgams have 'bonding' benefits:

- Less microleakage
- Less interfacial staining
- Slightly increased strength of remaining tooth structure
- Minimal post-operative sensitivity
- Some retention benefits

However, bonded amalgams are more technique-sensitive compared with conventional amalgam restorations.

3   Answer any questions they may have.

OSCE Station 4.9

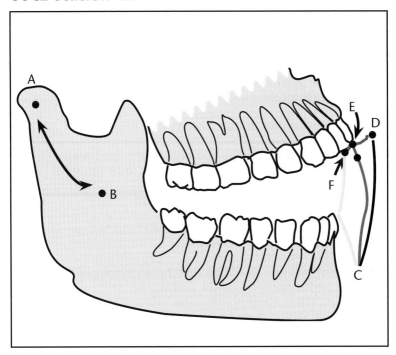

The yellow or the most posterior line indicates opening. The first part of the curve is a hinge movement with the condyles situated posteriorly in the fossae. After about 2.5 cm the mandibular condyles start to translate and the curve shifts anteriorly. Point C is maximum opening. The blue line represents closure from maximum opening with the mandible protruded, and point D is maximum protrusion in a closed position. The red line then follows the movement of the mandible from maximum protrusion in a closed position to intercuspal position (E) and then onward to retruded contact position (F). These are movements that would only be carried out consciously; normal patterns of movement are represented by the green line. Point A is the fulcrum of movement when simple hinge movements are made and point B is where the fulcrum shifts to during translatory movements of the mandible.

OSCE Station 4.10

1 Shake the powder bottle to ensure that the contents are mixed.

2 Fill the dispensing scoop.

3 Level the powder in the dispensing scoop by rubbing the scoop against the plastic lip of the bottle.

4 Place the powder on the mixing pad.

5 Dispense an appropriate number of even-sized drops (holding the bottle vertically will help drops to be of similar sizes).

6 Add the powder to the liquid in one go.

7 Mixing times vary depending on the brand but are usually between 30 and 45 seconds.

8 The final mixture should be stretchy, so that it can be stretched about 1 cm off the pad.

9 It should still be shiny when used – if it looks matt it has started to set.

10 Clean the spatula and mixing pad as soon as possible as the set material is hard to remove.

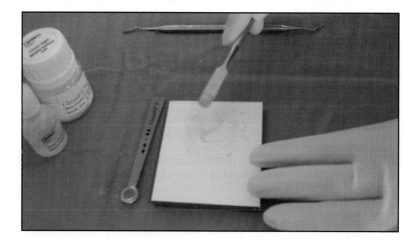

OSCE Station 4.11

1   Introduce yourself politely to the patient.

2   Explain to her the causes of intrinsic tooth discoloration and the treatment options available.

A   Causes of tooth discoloration:

- Amelogenesis imperfecta
- Dentinogenesis imperfecta
- Fluorosis
- Tetracycline staining
- Trauma
- Chronological hypoplasia
- Age changes
- Caries

B   Treatment options available:

- Vital bleaching.
- 'In surgery' bleaching – Use 30–35% carbamide or hydrogen peroxide. Dental curing light is often used to activate the bleaching agent.
- Home bleaching using a custom-made bleaching splint – Following fitting of the splint the patient uses carbamide peroxide (10%) for 6–8 hours treatment per day. They are kept under review to monitor the progress. Home bleaching techniques are easily applied and repeatable, but can be unpredictable with tetracycline staining. They are only appropriate when there are minimal or no restorations in the teeth.
- Non-vital bleaching – This allows bleaching of deeper dentine and has a greater effect on change in colour.
- Microabrasion with acid and pumice ± hydrogen peroxide.
- Composite resin veneers – Some tooth preparation is needed but is less destructive than crowns. When there is severe (dark) discoloration the tooth may need bleaching first. They provide a good result, but over time may shrink, stain and wear and so may need replacing after about 4 years.
- Porcelain veneers – About 0.5 mm of tooth substance is removed, but again this is less destructive than for crown preparation. They are constructed in the laboratory and

bonded onto the etched enamel surface. They provide better performance and aesthetic appearance and are less plaque-retentive than composite resin veneers.

- Crowns – These provide an excellent aesthetic appearance and are retentive and strong, but are destructive of tooth substance. They are a good option if the tooth is already heavily restored.

3   Answer any questions she may have.

OSCE Station 4.12

A

- Prefabricated or custom-made
- Parallel-sided or tapered
- Threaded, smooth or serrated

B

	Advantage	Disadvantage
Prefabricated	Cheap and quick	Less versatile and requires removal of all coronal dentine
Custom made	More versatile	Expensive, extra laboratory stage
Parallel-sided	Greater retention, generates less stress in root canal	More likely to perforate in apical region
Tapered	Less likely to perforate in apical region, better for small tapered roots	Less retention
Threaded	Greater retention compared with smooth sided post	Increased stress within root canal
Smooth	Less stress within root canal	Less retention compared with serrated or threaded
Serrated	Increased surface area for retention without concentration of stress	Increased stress within root canal

Table 4.12

OSCE Station 4.13

A

1   Introduce yourself politely to the patient.

2   Explain to the patient what you plan to do, ie test whether the tooth in question is still alive by applying a stimulus to it and gain their permission.

3   It is also useful to test adjacent teeth or the contralateral tooth as a control.

Vitality tests

Ethyl chloride test:

- This is the application of cold.
- Spray ethyl chloride onto a pledget of cotton wool and hold it against the tooth for several seconds or until a change in temperature is noted by the patient.

Gutta percha:

- This is the application of heat.
- Dry the tooth and apply petroleum jelly (Vaseline) to it, as this will stop the hot gutta percha from sticking to the tooth. Heat the gutta percha and apply to the tooth for a few seconds or until a response is noted by the patient.

Electric pulp tester:

- Dry the tooth and then apply the prophy paste.
- It is necessary to make a circuit, so, depending on the design of the machine, either the patient has to hold some part of the machine or you must touch the patient.
- Apply to the tip to the tooth at the lowest setting on the dial and slowly increase the power until the patient notes a response. (NB: the actual reading bears little resemblance to the state of the pulp as it can vary depending on the position it is applied to on the tooth or the amount of power in the battery.)

B

Possible causes of false positives:

- Multiple root canals containing vital and non-vital pulp at the same time
- Nervous patient
- Pus in canals

Possible causes of false negatives:

- Presence of a large restoration that insulates the pulp
- A vital pulp with a good blood supply but a damaged nervous supply (NB: pulp testing really tests the nervous stimulation of the pulp rather than its blood supply, which is of more importance in maintaining vitality)
- Secondary dentine insulating the stimulus reaching the pulp

OSCE Station 4.14

The appropriate method of isolation for endodontic treatment is application of a rubber dam. Other methods are considered negligent due to the risk of inhalation of instruments, so selecting the parachute chain is wrong.

1   Prior to commencement of the root canal treatment, punch holes in the dam to go over the tooth/teeth. For endodontic treatment it is only necessary to expose the tooth you are working on through the dam, although sometimes adjacent teeth may be exposed.

2   Select an appropriate clamp.

3   Apply a piece of floss to the clamp.

4   Either put the clamp and floss through the hole in the dam, apply clamp-holding forceps and place them all on the tooth together or put the clamp and floss on the tooth with the clamp-holding forceps and then stretch the dam over the seated clamp.

5   Floss the dam into the contact points and apply wedges if needed.

6   Place a piece of gauze beneath the rubber and the patient's skin.

7   Apply the frame.

8   Secure the loose floss to the frame.

OSCE Station 4.15

A

1 Attach the study model firmly to the cast table on the surveyor.

2 Orientate the occlusal plane at 90° to the base of the surveyor.

3 Place the analyser rod in the surveyor and gently run around the teeth present on the cast. Assess the study model for guide planes and undercuts where clasps could be used to gain retention. It may be necessary to tilt the cast to use some undercuts or even out others.

4 When the final angle of tilt has been decided, remove the analyser rod and replace with the carbon tip. Then run this around the cast to mark all the undercuts on hard and soft tissue alike.

B Study models are surveyed as part of the denture design process. Surveying involves locating the maximum contour of individual teeth, alveolar ridges and residual ridges. It is used to identify the path of insertion and withdrawal of the denture. Once this is known it is possible to identify which undercuts need to be blocked out. This will ensure that no part of a rigid denture will lie in an undercut relative to the path of insertion. It will also identify which undercuts can be left to aid retention of the denture, and the amount of horizontal undercut of the teeth selected for clasping can be determined. Surveying is important because it enables a denture to be designed with the easiest path of insertion, coupled with the greatest retention and resistance to displacement.

OSCE Station 4.16

1   Introduce yourself politely to the patient.

2   Patient's complaint – You need to ascertain the chief complaint and write it in the notes in the patient's own words.

3   History of present complaint:

   • Is this a new problem or have the teeth always had this appearance?
   • Did the deciduous teeth have a similar appearance?
   • Are there any associated features, such as pain or sensitivity?

4   Ask about possible factors, both environmental and genetic, which may be responsible, for example:

   • Trauma to teeth
   • Systemic infections/illness
   • Exposure to any toxic substances
   • Any high intake of fluoride/tetracycline as child
   • Any hereditary disorders.

5   Check the patient's medical history – Any systemic illness(es) and the age it occurred.

6   Ask the patient if he has any questions.

Comment

From the above history it should be possible to determine the likely cause of the dental appearance.

OSCE Station 4.17

A

The patient has horizontal bands of yellow/brown discoloration affecting his maxillary and mandibular incisors and canine teeth. It is not possible to see in this picture if his first molars are also affected. The most likely diagnosis is enamel hypoplasia, possibly the result of disturbance during the period of tooth development in childhood. The enamel is reduced in thickness or of deficient structure and may present as pits, linear or groove defect along enamel.

B

The management of intrinsic staining may be difficult, and depending on severity, the restorative options are:

- Tooth bleaching and micro-abrasion (this may be an option if the defect was localised and minimal)
- Veneers: composite/porcelain.
- Crowns (depending on the extent of tooth involvement).

Micro-abrasion

This is a procedure where a small amount of the stained tooth substance is removed by using a combination of an abrasive impregnated wheel and dilute acid.

- Advantage: No restorative material is used
- Disadvantage: Useful only if developmental problem or staining is fairly superficial (several hundred micrometres only).

Bleaching

This is the use of chemicals to lighten or whiten darken/discolored teeth.

- Advantage: No need for removal of tooth substance. No need for restorative material to be used.
- Disadvantage: Effect is not permanent. It will be of limited use in this case as the problem is not only staining, as there are also enamel defects to address. Bleaching can make teeth sensitive.

Veneers (ceramic/composite)

A veneer is a facing placed on the surface (labial in this case) of the tooth. This usually requires tooth preparation.

- Advantage: Veneers are effective for masking substantial hypoplastic enamel so would be suitable in this case.
- Disadvantage: The enamel thickness needs to be reduced by half on the labial surface. Requires acid etching. Very dark staining may not be masked by veneers.

Crowns (partial jacket crown and dentine-bonded crown)

A crown is a restoration ('cap') that encompasses (covers) the coronal tooth tissue (tooth tissue that is present above the gum).

- Advantage: Used when there is inadequate tooth structure to support a veneer. Can be used to mask darker staining. Good aesthetics.
- Disadvantage: Requires tooth preparation – more than required with veneers.

Comment

At the end of the discussion remember to ask if the patient has any questions.

Other aetiologies that may be considered are:

- Hereditary (amelogenesis or dentinogenesis imperfecta, porphyria)
- Acquired
  - Nutritional deficiencies
  - Infections
  - Trauma during dental development
  - Exposure to chemicals.

The cause/aetiology may also be sub-categorised into intrinsic and extrinsic factors that cause tooth discoloration.

Intrinsic factors:

- Amelogenesis imperfecta
- Dentinogenesis imperfecta
- Porphyria

- Fluorosis
- Tetracycline staining
- Enamel hypoplasia
- Neonatal jaundice
- Non-vitality and root filling.

Extrinsic factors:

- Mouthwashes
- Discolored restorations
- Tea, coffee, red wine
- Smoking.

OSCE Station 4.18

1   Before the patient arrives into the clinic, the crown should be checked on the model. Things to look at are:

- The contact points
- The occlusion with opposing teeth
- The die and adjacent teeth for rub marks
- Check there are no blobs of cast metal on the fit surface, if there are, these need to be ground down.
- NB: if it was a ceramic crown you would also check the shade but this is not necessary in this case.

2   When the patient arrives:

(a) Check that there is no change in their medical history since the last visit.
(b) Check that the patient has not had any problems with the tooth in question since the last visit.
(c) Give a local anaesthetic if required. However, remember that a local anaesthetic may alter the patient's perception of the occlusion.

3   Remove the temporary crown from the lower left first molar. Clean the preparation to remove all traces of cement.

4   Try in the restoration, you may need to check the contacts with floss to help it to seat.

5   Check the margins of the crown: there should be no overhangs and there should be a smooth transition from restoration to tooth.

6   Check the gingival emergence profile.

7   Check the occlusion. Using fine articulating paper is better as thick paper will not differentiate between normal occlusal stops and high points. It is easier to see minor irregularities if the surface of the restoration is not extremely shiny. Static occlusion and dynamic occlusion must both be checked. High spots and heavy contacts must be removed but care must be taken not to make the remaining restoration too thin.

8   Cement the tooth:

  (a) The prepared surface of the tooth should be cleaned
       and dried.
  (b) The fit surface of the crown should be cleaned and dried.
  (c) The cement should be placed around the fit surface of
       the crown.
  (d) The crown should be seated on the preparation with
       considerable pressure, which will expel excess cement.
  (e) The pressure should be maintained until the cement
       has set.
  (f) Excess cement should be flicked away from the margin
       and contact areas should be cleared with floss.

9   Recheck the occlusion.

10   Arrange a review.

OSCE Station 4.19

1   Introduce yourself politely to the patient.

2   Ascertain if the missing teeth were ever present in mouth.
     If they were never present you will need to carry out further
     investigations to determine that the tooth is unerupted (NB:
     absent maxillary lateral incisors are hereditary in 1–2% of
     the population).

3   Extra oral examination – Check the smile line. Does patient
     show any gingival/alveolus?

4   Intra-oral examination – Check the health of oral mucosa.
     Do a periodontal assessment: oral hygiene, any calculus,
     pocketing, gingival inflammation.

5   Assess the ridge height and width, and bone quality and
     quantity. To accommodate a standard implant there should
     be a minimum of 10 mm bone inciso-gingivally and a
     minimum of 6 mm facio-lingually. (NB: short and narrow
     implants are commercially available).

6   Assess the occlusion.

7   Special investigations

     •   Vitality testing of adjacent teeth to ensure no further
         treatment is required as they may be used as abutments.
     •   Radiographs – assess for unerupted teeth, pathology.
         •   Periapical or standard upper occlusal.
         •   DPT is helpful in the assessment of the overall
             dentition and to assess if there is adequate space
             between the roots to accommodate an implant.
     •   Study models for occlusal assessment and diagnostic
         wax-up.
     •   Clinical photographs.

8   Management of these patients may require a multi-
     disciplinary approach that may include an orthodontist,
     dental implantologist and restorative dentist.
     The options for treatment include closure of space by
     orthodontic means or a restorative option with
     maintenance of the space.

Closure of space by orthodontic means

- Complete space closure – Reshape the canine to resemble the lateral incisor.

    - Advantage: No need for fixed prosthesis.
    - Disadvantages: Disguising a canine to resemble a lateral incisor is rarely ideal (the tooth will still look bulky and prominent). Also, long treatment time compared with a restorative option.

- Partial space closure (as too much space for a lateral incisor).

    - Advantages: Allows correct size fixed prosthesis. Good aesthetics.
    - Disadvantage: Requires both orthodontic and restorative treatment, ie cost implications.

Restorative options with maintenance of space

- Fixed restoration: Fixed-fixed adhesive bridge (resin bonded).

    - Advantages: Minimal or no tooth preparation (conservative). Good aesthetics. Less chairside time and less expensive than a conventional bridge.
    - Disadvantages: Requires sound aesthetic abutment, and pontic retainer space is critical.
    No trial cementation. Requires adequate occlusal clearance. There is a risk of debonding of retainer, improved with more retentive designs. The retainer may affect the colour of the abutment teeth.

- Cantilever design

    - Advantages: Conservative, minimal tooth preparation. Good aesthetics and easy plaque control.
    - Disadvantages: Leverage on abutment teeth. If abutment debonds the patient is left with a space.

- Conventional bridge

    - Advantage: Fixed, good retention. Good aesthetic. Less sensitive cementation technique compared with resin-bonded.
    - Disadvantage: Greater tooth preparation, risk of pulp death. Failure due to decementation, decay of abutment teeth. Cost Irreversible. Requires temporary restoration

- Single tooth implant

    - Advantages: Fixed restoration. Independent of adjacent teeth for retention. Good maintenance of supporting bone.
    - Disadvantages: Requires adequate bone and involves a surgical procedure. High initial expense and long treatment time.

9   Ask if the patients has any questions and allow time for them to consider the options.

ORAL AND MAXILLOFACIAL SURGERY

Chapter 5: Questions

OSCE Station 5.1
5 minute station

You are a dentist working at 'Smiles Dental Practice', Borough End Road, Thamestown.

A 72-year-old man attends your surgery complaining of soreness on his tongue. This has been present for 4 weeks. There is no history of trauma to the tongue, and he is fit and healthy. On examination:
- There are no extra-oral abnormalities.
- There is an ulcer, 1 cm in diameter, on the right lateral border of the tongue.
- Teeth present are:

CHAPTER 5
Questions

6 4 3 2 1	1 2 3 4 5
7 4 3 2 1	1 2 3 6

Table 5.1

- There is a fractured amalgam restoration in the lower right second permanent molar.

A What factors would you ask about while taking the patient's social history?

B What initial management would you carry out for this patient?

C What features of the ulcer would lead you to suspect that it may be malignant?

D If the lesion is thought to be malignant, which type of biopsy should be taken?

OSCE Station 5.2
10 minute station

You are a dentist working at 'Smiles Dental Practice', Borough End Road, Thamestown.

The patient in Station 5.1 has returned a fortnight after your initial management of the ulcer, ie removal of the sharp edge of the broken-down lower right second permanent molar. The ulcer is unchanged in character; it is still 1 cm in diameter with raised rolled edges.

Please write a referral letter for the patient to see a specialist for management of the lesion. Patient details are as follows:

Mr Thomas Smith
Date of birth: 13 August 1933
Address: 54 Burntash Avenue, Thamestown AB18 4CD.

Tel: 020 7123 9876

OSCE Station 5.3
5 minute station

Please obtain consent from this patient for the removal of the lower right first permanent molar under local anaesthesia and intravenous sedation.

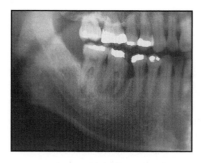

OSCE Station 5.4
5 minute station

You have just carried out forceps extraction of a lower right first permanent molar under local anaesthesia. Please give post-operative instructions to this patient.

OSCE Station 5.5
5 minute station

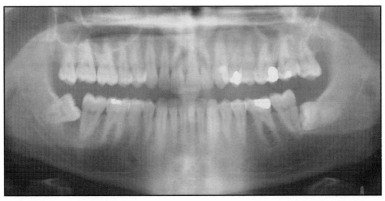

This patient requires the removal of both lower wisdom teeth.

Please warn them of the possible complications of removing these teeth.

OSCE Station 5.6
5 minute station

You are an SHO working in an oral and maxillofacial surgery department. You are seeing a fit and healthy 23-year-old lady who requires surgical removal of all four wisdom teeth due to multiple episodes of pericoronitis. The patient is unsure whether she could cope with the procedure under local anaesthesia and wants to know if there are any other ways in which the teeth could be removed, and what these would involve. Please explain to the patient what options are available to control pain and anxiety during surgical procedures.

OSCE Station 5.7
5 minute station

You are a dentist in general practice and are seeing an emergency patient, a 40-year-old with insulin-dependent diabetes, who has presented with an extra-oral swelling caused by a dental abscess from a carious lower right first permanent molar.

A   What clinical findings would lead you to believe that this patient has a rapidly spreading infection?

B   What criteria would you use for deciding whether to refer the patient on for treatment and who would you refer the patient to?

OSCE Station 5.8

5 minute station

You are a dentist in general practice. This fit and healthy patient has attended your surgery with pain in their upper right second molar. The patient is not keen to undergo further restorative work and wishes to have the tooth removed. A radiograph of the tooth is shown below.

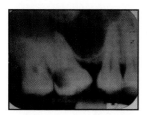

Please explain to the patient what removing the tooth under local anaesthetic involves, including possible complications.

OSCE Station 5.9
5 minute station

You are an SHO in an oral and maxillofacial surgery department. You are seeing a 25-year-old woman who you have diagnosed as suffering from myofascial pain in their masticatory system. Please give her advice on how she can manage the condition conservatively.

OSCE Station 5.10
5 minute station

A   Please select a suitable suture to use in an intra-oral wound.

B   Select some suitable instruments and place a single interrupted suture across the wound in this suture board.

Props:

- Variety of sutures
- Needle holders
- Clips
- Variety of forceps, toothed and non-toothed
- Variety of scissors, blunt-ended and sharp
- Suture board

a

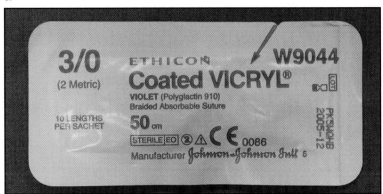

b

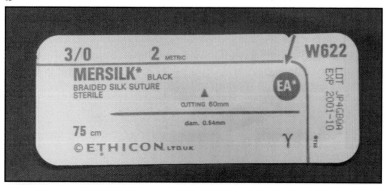

c

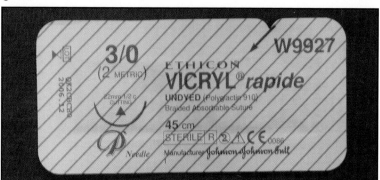

d

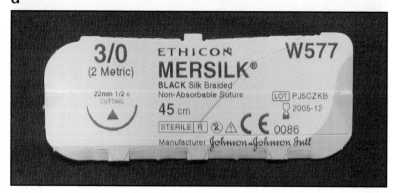

e

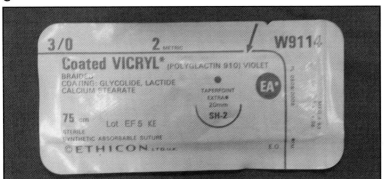

f

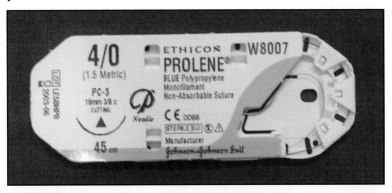

g

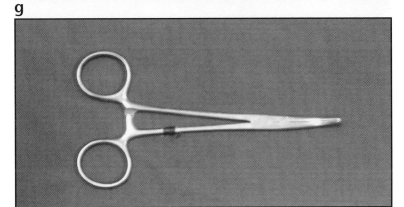

h

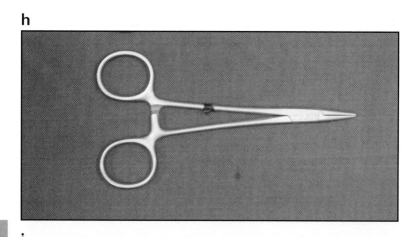

i

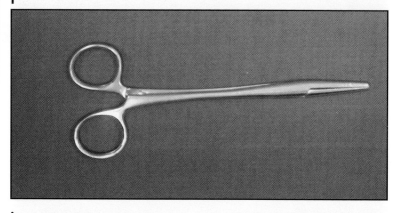

j

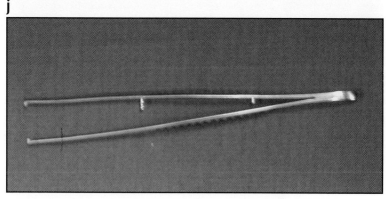

k

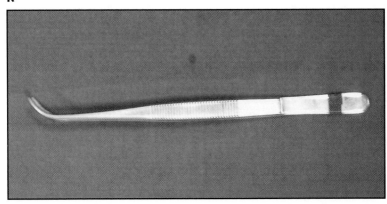

l

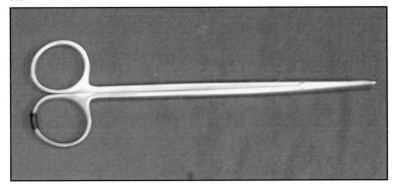

m

n

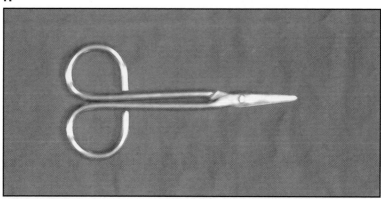

o

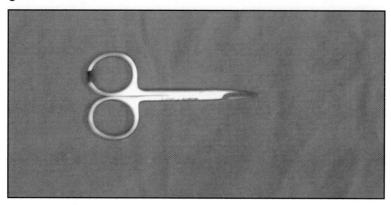

OSCE Station 5.11
5 minute station

You are a maxillofacial SHO and have been called to see a patient who has a bilateral dislocation of the temporomandibular joints (TMJs). Describe how you would proceed to reposition the mandible.

OSCE Station 5.12
5 minute station

Please name these instruments and indicate what they would be used for.

a

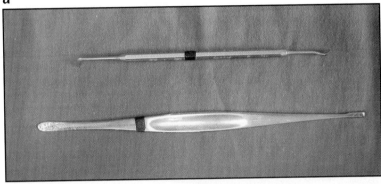

b

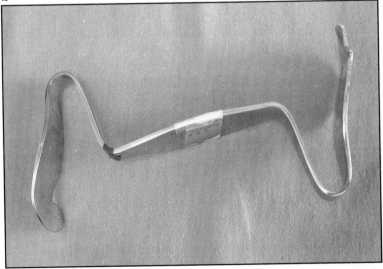

c

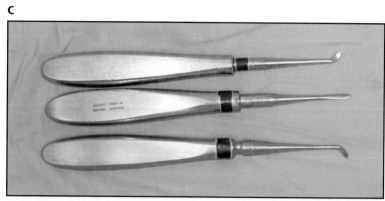

d

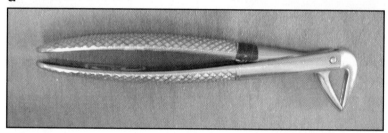

e

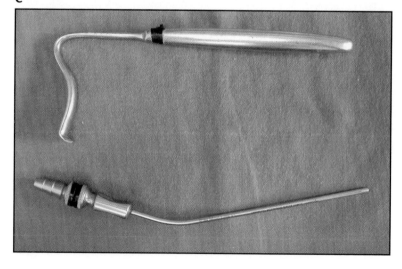

f

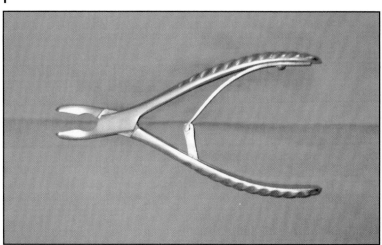

g

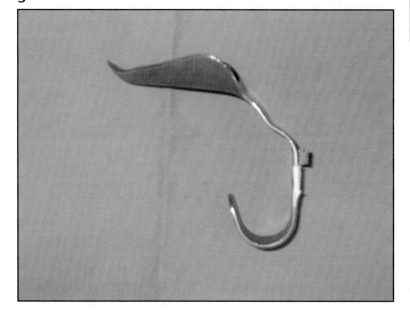

h

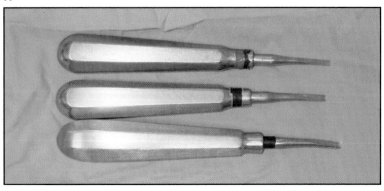

OSCE Station 5.13
5 minute station

These three lines describe paths of opening of the mandible as measured from the tip of the central incisors when looking at the patient from the front.

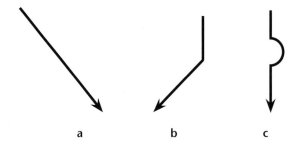

a   b   c

A   What is happening in the TMJs to account for the different lines of opening?

B   You want to ask a patient to carry out retruded jaw opening exercises. Please explain to them how to do these exercises.

OSCE Station 5.14
5 minute station

You are a dentist in general practice and seeing a patient who is complaining of pain in the lower second premolar. Examination reveals that the tooth is root treated and has a post crown restoration on it. Radiographs reveal a periapical radiolucency associated with the root.

Please explain to the patient what the various treatment options are for this tooth.

OSCE Station 5.15
5 minute station

A fit and healthy 24-year-old woman attends your surgery complaining of a clicking jaw joint, although this is not associated with any pain. This has been occurring over the past few years, but recently she has noticed that sometimes her jaw locks and she cannot open it. Please explain to her what could be happening to cause these symptoms.

OSCE Station 5.16
5 minute station

You are an SHO in an oral surgery unit seeing new patients on a consultation clinic. Mr Cooke, a 65-year-old man, has been referred in to your unit for removal of a lower second molar under local anaesthesia. Mr Cooke has prosthetic heart valves and takes warfarin 5 mg daily. His INR was 2.6 when it was checked 7 days ago. Please explain what pre-operative tests or measures are needed to manage Mr Cooke with regard to his prosthetic heart valves and warfarin usage.

OSCE Station 5.17
5 minute station

A patient in your practice requires removal of the upper left wisdom tooth. The procedure is straight forward but the patient is demanding that it is done under general anaesthesia. How will you manage this situation?

OSCE Station 5.18
5 minute station

How do you do the following sutures and when would you use them?

1 Continuous suture
2 Vertical mattress
3 Horizontal mattress

Chapter 5: Answers

OSCE Station 5.1

A Details regarding smoking and alcohol intake need to be ascertained, as well as other high-risk activities such as betel-nut chewing and snuff usage.

B Initial management would involve removing any local cause of irritation to the tongue to exclude a traumatic cause for the ulcer. The lower second permanent molar with the fractured amalgam restoration therefore needs to be treated. The restoration could be smoothed, or replaced with either a temporary or a permanent restoration so long as this leaves no sharp edges against the tongue, or even extracted.

C A malignant ulcer has raised rolled edges, and it is firm to the touch.

D A malignant ulcer should undergo incisional biopsy. This is because the surgeon who eventually comes to treat the lesion will be able to see where it is. If it is removed by an excisional biopsy there will be no lesion for the surgeon to see.

OSCE Station 5.2

Points to remember when writing the referral letter:

- The letter should be addressed to a consultant in oral and maxillofacial surgery.
- It must be marked urgent.
- It must include your contact details, ie address and telephone number.
- It must include the patient's contact details, ie address and telephone number.
- It must include a brief summary of the problem, treatment carried out and a provisional diagnosis.

A sample letter is shown below:

> Dr AN Other
> Smiles Dental Practice
> 21 Borough End Road
> Thamestown AB1 2CD
> Tel: 020 7123 4567
>
> Mr Chopper
> Department of Oral and Maxillofacial Surgery
> Thamestown General Hospital
> High Street
> Thamestown AB3 4CD
>
> **Re: Mr Thomas Smith, DOB. 13 August 1933**
> **54 Burntash Avenue, Thamestown AB18 4CD; Tel: 020 7123 9876**
>
> Dear Mr Chopper,
> I would be most grateful if you could see and treat Mr Smith urgently. He presented to the practice two weeks ago complaining of a sore area on his tongue which had been present for four weeks.
>
> Examination revealed no palpable neck nodes. Intra-orally there was a 1-cm- diameter ulcer on the right side of the tongue adjacent to a broken-down lower second permanent molar. I placed a temporary restoration in the tooth to prevent any further trauma to the area.
>
> *cont...*

At review today the ulcer is still present and in fact appears to have raised rolled margins. I am suspicious that the ulcer may be a squamous-cell carcinoma of the right side of the tongue.

Mr Smith is medically fit and healthy. He smokes 20 cigarettes a day and has done so for 40 years. He admits to being a social drinker, having approximately 10–12 pints of beer a week.

With kind regards
Yours sincerely

Dr AN Other

Note – some regions may have rapid access forms ie 2-week rule referral forms.

CHAPTER 5
Answers

OSCE Station 5.3

Points to cover are given below.

Local anaesthesia and sedation

- Explain that the patient will be awake and able to maintain verbal contact at all times.
- They will feel light-headed and perhaps a bit sleepy, and not anxious or worried by what is going on.
- The sedative agent is administered through a cannula, usually in the back of their hand.
- The local anaesthetic will have to be given inside their mouth because sedation will not numb the area.
- For the sedative agent to be administered they must attend with an escort, who is a competent adult, who will take them home and keep an eye on them for the remainder of the day.
- They should not drive or operate machinery or sign any legally binding documents in the next 24 hours. They should not eat for 2 hours prior to the procedure. If sedation is being administered by an anaethetist they prefer the patient to be starved as for a general anaesthetic.

The extraction

- The patient will not feel pain during the procedure but may be aware of pushing and pressure.
- The tooth may come out in one piece with forceps, or it may require a surgical approach. If so, a cut will be made in the gum, some bone may be removed from the wall of the socket, and the tooth may be cut into pieces to get it out.
- The patient will not feel any pain as the area will already be numb.
- Stitches will then be put into the gum.

Post-operatively

- It will be a bit sore and swollen.
- They may experience some bleeding from the extraction site afterwards, but instructions on care will be given after the procedure.
- They may experience limited mouth opening, and should be on a soft diet for several days.
- They may require antibiotics after the procedure.

OSCE Station 5.4

1   Introduce yourself politely to the patient.

2   You should give written and verbal instructions to patients following operative procedures. Points to cover:

- No rinsing of their mouth for about six hours as this may disturb the clot and cause bleeding from the socket.
- If bleeding does occur they should bite on a clean handkerchief (not a tissue) for 15 minutes. Pressure from biting should stop the bleeding.
- If bleeding cannot be controlled by biting on the handkerchief for 15 minutes, then the patient should contact you or an appropriate person.
- You need to give the patient details of how to contact someone for help should the bleeding not subside.
- Advise the patient on oral hygiene for the next few days. Warm, salty mouthwashes (put a teaspoon of salt in a glass of warm water) are ideal for keeping the socket clean and aiding healing. These should not be started until 6 hours after the procedure for fear of dislodging the clot.
- Advise them that mouthwashes are an adjunct to toothbrushing and should not be done instead of toothbrushing. Also mention that they may not be able to clean effectively round the socket with their toothbrush due to discomfort and this is where the mouthwashes are useful. Mouthwashes need to be used until the patient is able to clean well around the area with a brush.
- Pain relief – Advise the patient about suitable analgesics for the procedure. Forceps extraction of a tooth is not usually as uncomfortable as a surgical procedure, but patients may experience pain. Paracetamol 1 g four times a day is a good regimen, or if stronger pain relief is needed it can be combined with ibuprofen 400 mg three times a day (so long as there is nothing in the patient's medical history, such as asthma or peptic/gastric ulceration to contraindicate it).
- Advise the patient that they will still feel numbness following the procedure for a couple of hours so it is better for them to take an analgesic prior to the anaesthetic wearing off.
- Some degree of post-operative pain is to be expected. Severe pain that is worsening is abnormal, however, and advise the patient to contact you or an appropriate person if that happens.

- Warn the patient not to bite their lip while it is numb.
- Advise the patient that they can eat and drink after the procedure, but that they should avoid hot and chewy foodstuffs as these may cause the socket to bleed and will be difficult to eat.
- Advise the patient that some degree of swelling and limited mouth-opening is normal and should resolve in a few days.

3   Answer any questions they may have.

OSCE Station 5.5

1   Introduce yourself politely to the patient.

2   Points to cover:

- The patient needs to be warned that any extraction is usually accompanied by some degree of:
  - pain,
  - swelling,
  - post-operative bleeding, and
  - limited mouth-opening (trismus) after the procedure.

- They should be told what the procedure will entail:
  - Surgical procedure, with a cut being made in the gum, some bone of the socket being removed, the tooth being cut into pieces, and the gum stitched back into place afterwards.
  - Enucleation of any associated cystic tissue which would be sent for pathological examination.

- They should also be warned of specific complications associated with these extractions:
  - Numbness and tingling of lower lip and tongue – short-term and permanent.
  - Prognosis of lower second molars as there will be distal bone loss around these teeth.

- As the extractions may be difficult the patient may need time off work/college.

3   Answer any questions that they may have.

OSCE Station 5.6

1 Introduce yourself politely to the patient.

2 Points to cover are given below.

General anaesthesia

- The patient will be asleep while the procedure is carried out so she will not be aware of what is going on at all.
- The anaesthetic is usually administered through a cannula in the arm, so she may feel a sharp scratch as the cannula is inserted.
- She will need to allow some recovery time – several days off work/college.
- She will need to come in with an escort.
- She should not drive, sign legally binding documents, or operate any machinery for 24 hours.
- She will need to fast (starve) for 6 hours pre-operatively.
- She may feel nauseous and vomit after the procedure.
- Usually done as a day-case procedure, so she does not stay overnight in hospital.
- Modern anaesthetics are safe, but no anaesthetic is entirely without risk, so general anaesthesia should be avoided wherever possible. It is estimated that the risk of death is about 1:100 000.

Local anaesthesia with intravenous sedation

- She will be awake throughout the procedure. However, the sedation will mean that she will not be worried or anxious. It will make her feel drowsy and a bit drunk. It also has an amnesic effect so she probably will not remember the procedure.
- She will need to come in with an escort.
- She should not drive, sign legally binding documents, or operate any machinery for 24 hours.
- She will need to fast for 2 hours pre-operatively (although if sedation is carried out by an anaesthetist they prefer the patient to be fasted as for a general anaesthetic).
- Recovery time is shorter.
- It is a safer procedure.
- The sedative agent is administered through a cannula in

the arm, so she may feel a sharp scratch as the cannula is inserted.
- She will still need an injection to numb the area in the mouth.

Oral sedation

- Tablet sedation is administered either at home or an hour before the procedure to help calm the patient.
- It is not as reliable as intravenous administration.

3   Answer any questions that they may have.

OSCE Station 5.7

Points to cover:

A

- People with diabetes are at more risk of infections. Odontogenic infections can progress rapidly in diabetic patients, especially if the diabetes is poorly controlled. Infections can alter diabetic control, leading to changes in blood sugar levels.
- Signs of a spreading infection:
    - Increasing pain
    - Rapidly increasing swelling
    - Fever
    - Increased pulse rate
    - Uncontrolled diabetes

- When to refer:
    - Raised temperature (>38°C)
    - Increased pulse rate
    - Abnormal blood glucose levels
    - Raised floor of mouth
    - Firm floor of mouth
    - Drooling
    - Deviated uvula
    - Severe trismus
    - Difficulty swallowing
    - Inability to speak in complete sentences

B

- Refer to an oral and maxillofacial surgery department by contacting the SHO/specialist registrar or consultant.

OSCE Station 5.8

1   Introduce yourself politely to the patient.

2   Points to cover:

- The area will be numbed with local anaesthetic.
- The procedure will be painless but the patient may experience sensations of pressure and pushing.
- The tooth may come out with forceps in one piece. However, there is a large carious area so the tooth could fracture.
- The tooth may need to be removed surgically, which would involve a cut in the gum, bone removal, and possible cutting of the tooth into pieces to remove it. This would be followed by stitching of the gum.
- The maxillary sinus is visible on the radiograph and close to the root so there is a possibility that removing the tooth may create a communication between the mouth and the sinus. If this is a very small hole it may close with no surgical intervention. However, larger communications will need surgical closure – otherwise food and drink will enter the sinus and come out of the patient's nose while eating and drinking.
- Closure can be carried out as soon as the tooth is removed if a communication is noted, by stitching the gum across the hole.
- The patient will then have to avoid blowing their nose for 2 weeks.
- They may need antibiotics, nasal inhalations and nose drops post-operatively.
- There will be pain and swelling post-operatively.
- There will be limited mouth-opening post-operatively.
- The patient will have to take time off work/college.

3   Answer any questions that they may have.

OSCE Station 5.9

1   Introduce yourself politely to the patient.

2   Points to cover are given below.

Information

- Reassurance and explanation play a big role in the treatment of myofascial pain.
- Explain that the condition is very common, especially in young women.
- The exact cause is unknown although there are predisposing factors:
  - It is often stress-related, so worrying about it will make it worse.
  - Sometimes it is due to a discrepancy in bite or due to previous trauma.
  - Sometimes it is related to parafunctional activities such as nail-biting, chewing pen and pencil tops, clenching and grinding of teeth.

- The condition is usually self-limiting, although it may take months to years to resolve.
- Explain that her pain is coming from the muscles that move her jaw, which will get worse during use.

Treatment

- Explain that the treatment will take many forms and will take a while to work.
- The important point is to rest her jaw as much as possible.
- She should eat soft food. It does not have to be soup, although in acute episodes this may be ideal. Foods such as mashed potato, scrambled egg, ice cream, yoghurt are soft foods.
- She should limit mouth-opening – stifle a yawn with a fist under her mouth, for example.
- She should rest her jaw as much as possible, limit parafunctional habits – no chewing gum, no biting nails, no chewing pen tops.
- She should apply heat to the side of her face with a warm hot-water bottle.
- Prescribe non-steroidal anti-inflammatory drugs

(NSAIDs), provided these are not contraindicated by her medical history.

- Arrange a follow-up appointment to monitor her progress and advise her that if these simple measures are not helping there are other things you can do, such as making a soft bite-raising appliance and giving her retruded jaw exercises to carry out.

3 Answer any questions that she may have.

OSCE Station 5.10

A   The correct sutures to use here would be either 'c' (Vicryl®
rapide; resorbable) or 'd' (black silk; non-resorbable). Both
these are 3-0 sutures on curved cutting needles of an appropriate size. The others are:

(a)   3-0 Vicryl® ties

(b)   3-0 black silk suture on a straight needle

(e)   3-0 Vicryl® suture on a round-bodied needle

(f)   4-0 Prolene® suture

B   Choose the following instruments:

- Needle holder (h)
- Toothed tissue forceps (j)
- Scissors with a blunt end (m)

The others are:
- Curved clip (g)
- Straight clip (i)
- College forceps (k)
- Non-toothed forceps (l)
- Disposable scissors (n)
- Sharp dissecting scissors (o)

Then:

1   Mount the needle correctly in the needle holder.

2   Insert the needle at right angles to the tissue/wound edges.

3   Collect the needle.

4   Tie a careful reef knot, by looping the long end of the suture
around the needle holder twice, grasping the short end of
suture with the needle holder and pulling through.

5   Then form another loop of suture around the needle holder
in the opposite direction, grasp the short end of the suture
with needle the holder and pull through.

6   Repeat of the first step again, but with only one loop around the needle holder.

7   Tighten the knot.

8   Cut sutures ends – about 0.5 cm long.

9   Position the knot at one side of wound. If the knot does not lie to one side of the wound, then reposition it to one side.

OSCE Station 5.11

Reduction of dislocated TMJs can be carried out manually. It may be necessary to augment the treatment with local anaesthesia, sedation, or, in difficult cases, general anaesthesia.

1   Introduce yourself politely to the patient.

2   Explain to the patient what you are about to do.

3   Warn the patient not to open their mouth immediately after the reduction as it is likely to redislocate.

4   Perform the reduction with the patient sitting in a chair or lying supine.

Patient sitting down

1   It is important that the head is supported while you carry out the manoeuvre.

2   Stand in front of the patient.

3   Place your thumbs on the external oblique ridge or occlusal surface of the lower molars. (If you place your thumbs on the lower occlusal surface be aware that the patient may bite on them as they close their mouth.)

4   Place your fingers under the patient's chin.

5   Apply pressure with your thumbs in a downward direction and with your fingers in an upward direction.

6   Do not attempt to relocate the jaw by pushing backwards.

7   You may find it easier to replace one side first and then the other.

8   Once relocated, continue upward pressure on the chin for about 1 minute to prevent the patient from opening their mouth.

9   Advise the patient to avoid wide mouth opening for 24 hours.

Patient supine

1   Position the trolley or bed such that the patient is lying at your waist height.

2   Stand behind the patient's head.

3   Position fingers and thumbs as for seated patient.

4   Apply pressure with your thumbs in the direction of the patient's feet and with your fingers occlusally.

5   Again, one side may be relocated before the other.

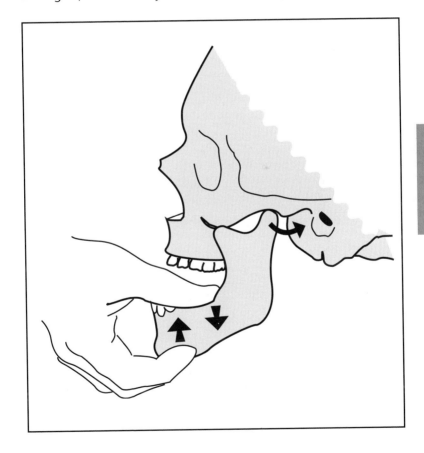

Additional measures, such as placement of a barrel bandage around the head and jaw or placement of a cervical collar, can be used to prevent redislocation in the immediate post-reduction phase.

If reduction alone is unsuccessful some additional measures may be employed:

- Sedation:
    - Intravenous midazolam
    - Nitrous oxide inhalation

- Local anaesthesia – around joint or into lateral pterygoid muscle
- General anaesthesia

OSCE Station 5.12

Instrument	Use
(a, top) Mitchell's trimmer	Curettage of soft tissues
(a, bottom) Howarth's periosteal elevator	Raising mucoperiosteal flaps, retracting periosteal flaps
(b) Ward's buccal retractor	Retracting periosteal flaps
(c) Warwick James elevators	Elevating teeth and roots
(d) Lower root forceps	Extracting lower anterior teeth
(e, top) Bowdler Henry Rake retractor	Retracting mucoperiosteal flaps
(e, bottom) American-style sucker	Aspirating blood and liquid from operating site
(f) Bone nibbler	Removing bone
(g) Laster's retractor	Retracting mucoperiosteal flaps when removing upper wisdom teeth
(h) Coupland's chisels	Elevating teeth and roots

Table 5.12

OSCE Station 5.13

A   (a) There are adhesions within the left TMJ, so when the patient opens the mouth the mandible deviates to the left as the left condyle is not able to translate. (b) There is a non-reducible obstruction within the right joint. Initially, opening is straight. Then the anteriorly displaced disc in the right TMJ prevents the right condyle from translating and the mandible deviates to the right. (c) There is a reducible obstruction within the TMJ. Opening starts straight and there is a deviation when the obstruction is encountered. However, the obstruction or the disc moves out of the way and so further opening is straight.

B   Retruded jaw opening exercises:

1   Introduce yourself politely to the patient.

2   Explain that the exercises are like physiotherapy for the jaw and need to be done regularly. Initially, ten times each in the morning, at lunchtime, in the evening and at night is a good regimen.

3   Advise them to do the exercises in front of the mirror initially.

4   Ask them to curl the tip of their tongue to the back of their hard palate this will get the mandible into a retruded position.

5   With the tongue in that position ask the patient to open and close their mouth slowly.

6   Ensure that they do not deviate to one side on opening, hence the need to sit in front of a mirror.

7   Ask them to repeat the manoeuvre so you are sure they can do the exercises.

OSCE Station 5.14

1 Introduce yourself politely to the patient.
2 Explain the treatment options as given below.

Procedure	Advantages	Disadvantages
Redo the root filling	Best option to get a good apical and coronal seal	The root may be fractured while removing the post crown to redo the root canal filling.
		May not be able to remove the post
		May not be able to improve on the previous root canal filling
		Multiple visits
Apicectomy and retrograde root filling	Reduces risk of fracture of the root as the post crown does not have to be removed.	Surgical procedure with associated pain and discomfort. Surgical procedure will be undertaken close to the mental foramen with possible damage to mental nerve.
	Single visit surgical procedure	Does not provide as good a seal as a conventional orthograde root filling
		May not work as it may be the coronal seal that has caused the root canal filling to fail, in which case a new coronal restoration would be still needed
		Shortening of the root
Extraction	Quick and easy way to relieve the symptoms and cure the problem	No tooth after procedure
Do nothing and treat with antibiotics	Easy option	Does not treat the cause and the problem will reoccur

Table 5.14

3 Ask the patient if they have any questions.

OSCE Station 5.15

Clicking temporo-mandibular joints are very common among the general population.

1   Introduce yourself politely to the patient.

2   Describing the anatomy of the joint often helps:

 (a)   Explain that between the head of the jaw bone (condyle) and the socket (temporal bone) there is a cartilaginous disc within the joint.
 (b)   The disk of cartilage is supposed to be closely associated with the condyle but sometimes it becomes a bit loose and usually lies anterior to the condyle.

3   Explain that in this situation when moving the jaw, the condyle moves but the disc does not, so pressure builds up as the condyle tries to move under the disc. Suddenly the pressure is too great and the disc rapidly moves back to overlie the condyle.

4   Explain that this movement creates a popping or clicking noise that patients feel and hear. In some instances the condyle is unable to get past the disc and this results in a lock.

5   Ask the patient if they have any questions.

Comment

Painless clicking usually does not merit any treatment. Locking will merit treatment depending on how frequently it occurs, and what the patient wants. Treatment can vary from simple conservative management with jaw rest and a soft diet, exercises in retruded position and occlusal appliances to invasive joint procedures such as arthrocentesis, arthroscopy and open temporo-mandibular joint surgery.

OSCE Station 5.16

1   You should discuss the following points with the patient.

Warfarin usage

- Taking warfarin will make Mr Cooke more likely to experience haemorrhage during and after the extraction. However, the risk of thrombo-embolism after temporary withdrawal of warfarin treatment greatly outweighs the risk of bleeding following a tooth extraction. Therefore Mr Cooke should not stop his warfarin prior to a dental extraction.
- However, you can only carry out an extraction if you know the patient's INR. This should be measured no more than 72 hours before the extraction. It will involve a blood test, either a finger prick test that gives an instant result or a conventional blood test that will usually take 30 minutes to an hour before the result is back from the laboratory. The type of test carried out depends on the equipment available. If the INR is less than 4.0 then it is acceptable to remove the tooth. If the INR is greater than 4 the extraction will have to be rescheduled and the patient should be referred to the anticoagulation service. Mr Cooke will need a repeat INR as his last one was 7 days ago.
- Ideally schedule the extraction for early in the day and ideally early in the week so that any post-operative bleeding problems can be dealt with during the working day and week. It is common practice to pack the extraction socket with a haemostatic agent and place sutures to aid haemostasis.
- It is also necessary to give good, clear post-operative instructions on mouth care and what to do if bleeding occurs. Instructions about taking appropriate analgesics (not NSAIDs) should also be given. If antibiotics are prescribed, care must be taken to ensure that they do not interfere with warfain, eg metronidazole should be avoided.

Prosthetic heart valves

- Having prosthetic heart valves puts Mr Cooke at a greater risk of getting infective endocarditis following certain dental procedures than a patient with healthy natural heart valves.
- However, in March 2008 guidelines changed regarding the need for antibiotic prophylaxis for infective endocarditis and dental treatment in the UK.
- NICE no longer recommends that patients are given antibiotic cover or pre-operative mouth washes.

2   Ask Mr Cooke if he has any questions.

Comment

For further information see the NICE website (www.nice.org.uk) or the National Patient Safety Agency website (www.npsa.nhs.uk).

OSCE Station 5.17

1   Introduce yourself politely to the patient.

2   Patient's complaint – You need to ascertain their chief complaint and write it in the notes in their own words.

3   If pain or infection is not present, it is often helpful to use this visit to establish rapport with the patient and gain their trust. Limit treatment to procedures that are reasonably comfortable for the patient or for relief of symptoms, eg examination, polish, temporary restoration.

4   Establish what the patient is anxious about – injection, loss of control, previous bad experience?

5   Try and address their fears, eg fear of local anaesthetic, tell them about topical anaesthetic gel. Tell the patient you will stop treatment if they raise their hand (allows sense of control).

6   Allow plenty of time for the appointment.

7   Discuss techniques which may be helpful:

- Relaxation techniques
- Distraction – ask them to think hard about something else, wiggle their toes, music, television
- Hypnotherapy
- Counselling is a way to deal with fear and anxiety
- Sedation (inhalational, oral and intravenous).

8   Discuss booking the patient for a treatment appointment, eg early appointment, quiet clinic time, longer treatment session.

9   Explain that it is a simple and quick procedure and very suitable for extraction using local anaesthetic.

10   If despite all this, the patient still request general anaesthesia for the extraction then discuss the risks and benefits of local versus general anaesthesia.

Risk – benefit/why general anaesthesia is not a good idea

Explain to the patient that GA is a procedure which is never without risk. Explain what the risks are.

Local anaesthesia	General anaesthesia
No special preparation, can eat and drink before procedure	Fasted for 6 hours
No loss of consciousness/awake	Loss of consciousness
No nausea or vomiting	Nausea and risk of vomiting
No special equipment	Need to be supported by medical equipment to breathe
Can work towards coping with anxiety	Does not help alleviate or work towards control of anxiety
Fewer agents used so less risk of allergic reaction	Risk of reaction to the anaesthetic agent
Much lower risk	Low risk of death
	Need intravenous access

Table 5.17

NB: Humphris (1999) reported that a large population of anxious dental patients (46.5%) can be treated with behavioural management.

OSCE Station 5.18

1   Check you have the appropriate instruments:

- Needle holder
- Toothed tissue forceps
- Scissors with a blunt end

2   Choose the appropriate suture depending on tissue to be suturing, ie skin or mucosa.

Suturing technique

The choice of suturing technique depends on the type and anatomic location of the wound, the thickness of the skin or mucosa, the degree of tension, and the desired cosmetic result.

- Continuous sutures: These are useful for long wounds in which wound tension has been minimised and in which approximation of the wound edges is good.
  - Advantages of the simple running suture include quicker placement and approximation of wound edges.
  - Disadvantages include the risk of wound breakdown if the suture material breaks and difficulty in making fine adjustments along the suture line. Also release of the wound, for example to drain a haematoma, would require removal of the whole line of suturing.
- Vertical mattress: These are used to evert the skin edges, permit greater closure strength and better distribution of wound tension.
- Horizontal mattress: These used to spread tension along the wound edges.

Continuous suture

The simple continuous suture is an uninterrupted series of simple interrupted sutures (see OSCE station 5.10).

1   Mount needle correctly in needle holder.

2   Insert needle at right angles to the tissue/wound edges.

3   Collect needle.

4   Tie a careful reef knot, by looping the long end of the suture around the needle holder (two times), grasping the short end of suture with the needle holder and pulling through.

5   Then form another loop of suture around the needle holder in the opposite direction, grasp the short end of suture with the needle holder and pull through.

6   Repeat the first step again, but with only one loop around the needle holder.

7   Tighten the knot.

8   Only cut the short suture end, ie the one without the needle attached.

9   Place a series of simple sutures in succession without tying or cutting the suture material after each pass.

10   Sutures should be evenly spaced, and tension should be evenly distributed along the suture line.

11   The line of stitches is completed by tying a reef knot after the last pass at the end of the suture line. To tie this final knot, use the last part of the simple suture as the short end and tie the reef knot, by looping the long end of the suture around the needle holder (two times), grasping the short end of suture with the needle holder and pulling through and complete knot as in point 5 and 6.

Continuous over and over sutures

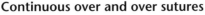

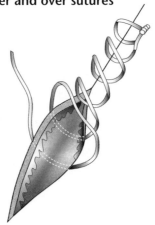

Horizontal mattress

The horizontal mattress suture is placed by entering the skin 5 mm to 1 cm from the wound edge. The suture is passed deep in the dermis to the opposite side of the suture line and exits the skin equidistant from the wound edge (in effect, a deep simple interrupted stitch). The needle re-enters the skin on the same side of the suture line 5 mm to 1 cm lateral to the exit point.

1 Mount needle correctly in needle holder.
2 Insert needle at right angles to the tissue/wound edges 4–8 mm from wound edges.
3 Pass the suture through to the opposite wound side and exit the skin equidistant from the wound edge.
4 Re-insert the needle in the skin on the same side, 4–8 mm further along the wound edge (that the needle has just passed through).
5 Pass the suture deep to the opposite side of the wound and exit the skin. Tie a knot (on the side of the wound where suturing began).

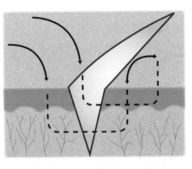

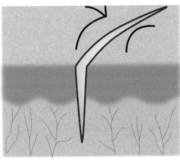

Vertical mattress

The vertical mattress suture is a variation of the simple interrupted suture. It consists of a simple interrupted stitch placed wide and deep into the wound edge and a second more superficial interrupted stitch placed closer to the wound edge and in the opposite direction.

6　Mount needle correctly in needle holder.

7　Insert needle at right angles to the tissue/wound edges for the far-far pass (further away from wound edge) 4–8 mm from wound edge

8　Now use the needle for the near-near pass, with the needle passing within 1–2 mm of the wound edges; the depth of this pass is superficial, ie 1–2 mm

9　Tie both ends of the suture on the same side of the wound.

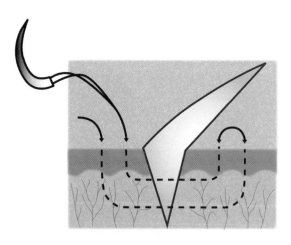

ORAL MEDICINE

Chapter 6: Questions

OSCE Station 6.1
10 minute station

You are a dentist in general practice. You are seeing a new patient who is a smoker and has smoker's keratosis. Please give the patient advice on stopping smoking.

OSCE Station 6.2
5 minute station

You are a dentist in general dental practice. A patient attends your surgery complaining of recurrent oral ulcers. Examination reveals minor aphthous ulcers. Please give this patient advice on aphthous ulcers.

OSCE Station 6.3
5 minute station

Which antimicrobial would you prescribe in the following clinical situations?

Condition	Antimicrobial of first choice	Alternative choice
Acute periapical abscess or periodontal abscess		
Acute ulcerative gingivitis		
Angular cheilitis		——————
Denture stomatitis		——————
Recurrent herpes labialis		
Primary herpetic gingivostomatitis		——————

Table 6.3a

OSCE Station 6.4
5 minute station

A patient attends your practice complaining of a dry mouth.

A   What are the possible causes of dry mouth?

B   What dental complications do patients with dry mouths suffer from?

OSCE Station 6.5
5 minute station

You are seeing a patient with a dry mouth in the oral medicine clinic. You suspect they have Sjögren's syndrome. You wish to carry out some special tests to confirm your diagnosis. Explain to the patient which special tests you want to get done and what they involve.

OSCE Station 6.6
5 minute station

A patient attends your surgery complaining of a white patch in their mouth. He is concerned about it.

A   What is the differential diagnosis of the lesion?

B   What steps would you take to reach a diagnosis?

OSCE Station 6.7
5 minute station

A patient has presented at your practice with this unilateral lesion in their mouth, which is sore.

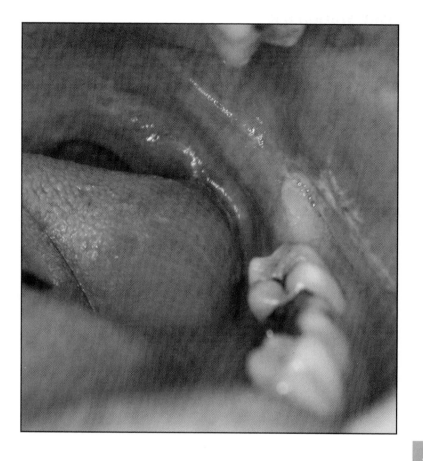

A What is the likely diagnosis?

B This condition can occur as one of a number of clinical subtypes. What are these?

C What are the predisposing factors?

D Where else can this condition occur and what are the lesions like?

OSCE Station 6.8
5 minute station

Please explain to the patient in Station 6.7 what lichen planus is and how you plan to manage it.

OSCE Station 6.9
5 minute station

This 24-year-old woman is complaining of recurrent cold sores on her lip. On examination, she has herpes labialis. Please explain to her what the sores are and how to manage them.

OSCE Station 6.10
5 minute station

Please obtain consent from this fit and healthy patient for the surgical removal of a fibroepithelial polyp from her tongue under local anaesthesia.

Prop:

- Consent form.

OSCE Station 6.11
10 minute station

Please carry out an excisional biopsy of this fibroepithelial polyp on this biopsy pad.

a

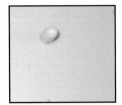

Props:

- Scalpel with no. 15 blade
- Toothed tissue forceps
- Needle holder
- 3-0 suture (black silk or Vicryl®)
- Suture scissors
- Biopsy pad

OSCE Station 6.12
5 minute station

You are reviewing a patient who has had an incisional biopsy for a white patch in their mouth. The histopathology report states that the lesion shows features of mild dysplasia. Please explain to the patient what this means, the significance of the diagnosis and how this may be managed.

Chapter 6: Answers

OSCE Station 6.1

Nowadays, the commonest method is the modified 'five As' approach:

- Ask – check smoking status
- Advise – value of quitting
- Assist – offer appropriate support
- Arrange – local smoking cessation service
- Assess

Ask

- Do they smoke?
- How many cigarettes do they smoke a day?
- How soon after waking do they smoke their first cigarette?
- Do they want to stop smoking for good?
- Are they interested in making a serious attempt to stop smoking in the near future?
- Are they interested in receiving help with their attempt to quit?

Advise

- Emphasise the fact that stopping smoking is the single most effective step they could take to improve their present state of health.
- Explain that past failures may actually improve their chances of quitting this time. People who keep trying to stop are more likely to give up in the end.
- Smokers often do not realise that smoking causes other diseases than lung cancer and heart disease, for example mouth cancer. This should be pointed out, with emphasis placed on oral health, eg mention halitosis, stained teeth, healthier gums and oral soft-tissues.

It has been estimated that smoking 20 cigarettes a day for the next 10 years would cost over £16 000 based on 2003 prices (Action on Smoking and Health).

Assist

- If during the previous two stages the patient expresses a desire to stop smoking, then help must be offered.
- Negotiate a stop date, which will allow them time to prepare.
- Review past attempts at quitting.
- Try to anticipate any potential problems.
- Suggest enlisting the help of family and friends.
- Advise them that nicotine replacement therapy is available.
- Tell them about the NHS Stop Smoking Service.

Arrange

- Tell the patient that you can arrange for them to be referred to the NHS Stop Smoking Service, where they can have one-to-one or group counselling sessions.
- Tell them that they can also refer themselves and give them the Helpline telephone number (0800 169 0169) or Quitline number (0800 002 200).
- Monitor their progress at future dental appointments and provide support and encouragement.

Assess

- Arrange follow-up.

OSCE Station 6.2

1 Introduce yourself politely to the patient.

2 Points to cover:

- Recurrent aphthous ulceration is a common mucosal disorder (~5–20% of the population are affected at some time in their lives).
- It is more common in females.
- No single causative factor has been identified.
- There is often a familial tendency.
- Alterations in some blood factors, such as reduced levels of iron, folic acid or vitamin B_{12} are found in up to 20% of patients. Correction of this deficiency results in resolution of the symptoms.
- There are some predisposing factors:
  - Hypersensitivity to foodstuffs, eg benzoate preservatives E210–219
  - Cessation of smoking
  - Psychological factors
  - Injury to the mucosa

- In some cases there is no identifiable cause.
- Diagnosis is based on the history and clinical features, and biopsy is not usually needed.
- Treatment is based on identifying predisposing factors and treating them, followed by symptomatic relief:
  - Blood tests are done to exclude haematinic deficiencies. This is extremely important if the patient has associated gastrointestinal symptoms, heavy menstrual blood loss or is a vegan. Blood tests should include a full blood count, levels of vitamin B_{12}, whole blood folate and ferritin levels.
  - Avoid foodstuffs containing benzoate preservatives (E210–219).
  - Avoid crisps and chocolate.

- For symptomatic relief:
  - Mouthwashes
    - Chlorhexidine
    - Sodium bicarbonate
    - Benzydamine
    - Tetracycline (250 mg tablet in water four times

daily for a week)
  - Doxycycline
- Topical steroids
  - Hydrocortisone
  - Triamcinolone
  - Beclometasone
  - Betamethasone

- Systemic treatment when severe, but to be prescribed only by a specialist:
  - Prednisolone
  - Monoamine oxidase inhibitors
  - Thalidomide
  - Dapsone
  - Levamisole

3   Answer any questions that they may have.

OSCE Station 6.3

Condition	Antimicrobial of first choice	Alternative
Acute periapical abscess or periodontal abscess	Amoxicillin 250–500 mg three times daily (5/7) Erythromycin 250–500 mg four times daily (5/7)	Metronidazole 200–400 mg three times daily (5/7)
Acute ulcerative gingivitis	Metronidazole 200–400 mg three times daily (5/7)	If patient is not able to take metronidazole consider penicillin
Angular cheilitis	Miconazole gel topically and either amphotericin B lozenges 10 mg four times daily (14/7) or Fluconazole 50 mg once daily (7–14/7)	
Denture stomatitis	Nystatin 100 000 units four times daily (7/7) Miconazole 5–10 ml of gel in mouth four times daily (10/7) Amphotericin B lozenges 10 mg four times daily (14/7) Fluconazole 50 mg once daily (7–14/7)	
Recurrent herpes labialis	Topical aciclovir 5% five times a day (5/7)	Aciclovir 200 mg five times a day (5/7) (systemic aciclovir usually indicated only if patient is immunocompromised or for cold sores that recur frequently)
Primary herpetic gingi-vostomatitis	Systemic aciclovir 100–200 mg five times a day (5/7)	

Table 6.3b

OSCE Station 6.4

A   Causes of dry mouth:

- Drug therapy (eg anticholinergics, antihistamines, anti-reflux agents, tricyclic antidepressants)
- Anxiety
- Radiation damage to salivary glands
- Immune-related diseases, eg Sjögren's syndrome
- Dehydration
- Diabetes
- Renal failure
- Congenital absence of glands is extremely rare

B   Patients do not usually have problems unless salivary function is reduced by more than 50%. The problems include:

- Difficulty talking and swallowing
- Altered taste
- Uncomfortable mouth
- Unretentive dentures
- Lack of saliva, leading to generalised erythema of the oral mucosa and a lobulated dorsum of the tongue
- Predisposition to infections of the oral cavity, including:
  - Angular cheilitis and oral candidiasis
  - Cervical caries
  - Recurrent caries around existing restorations
  - Episodes of suppurative sialadenitis

OSCE Station 6.5

1 Introduce yourself politely to the patient.

2 Explain the special tests you want to carry out.

Salivary flow rate

- Explain that you need to measure the rate of production of saliva in the mouth.
- One way is to collect mixed saliva from the whole mouth over a certain length of time. This involves collecting all the saliva produced by getting the patient to spit into a universal tube. This can be done at rest and after chewing a piece of wax to get a stimulated flow rate.
- The other way is to collect salivary from an individual salivary gland, eg to test parotid flow rate. Parotid salivary flow rate can be measured by using a Carlsson–Crittenden cup which is a small device that fits over the parotid duct orifice in the buccal vestibule. This can be done at rest or by stimulating the flow by placement of a dilute solution of citric acid on the tongue.

Ocular or eye tests

- Lacrimal gland flow rate by Schirmer's test – Explain that tear production is often decreased when salivary flow rate is decreased. This is the reason you wish to check it. It involves placing a piece of filter paper under the lower eyelid for 5 minutes and measuring how far the moisture travels along the paper. Less than 5 mm is indicative of reduced production of tears.
- Rose Bengal score – This involves placing a dye in the eye.

Labial gland biopsy

Explain that taking a sample from a small salivary gland from the lower lip can determine whether they are suffering from Sjögren's syndrome. It involves a small surgical procedure under local anaesthesia. An incision is made on the inside of the lower lip and some minor salivary gland tissue removed for histological examination. The area is sutured and it usually heals within a week. It will, however be a bit sore and swollen during the healing phase.

Sialography

Explain that this involves injecting a radio-opaque dye into a salivary gland duct and then taking radiographs of the gland and associated duct. This then shows the architecture of the gland and duct and any strictures, stones or filling defects will be seen, along with functional abnormalities of the gland.

Scintigraphy

Explain that this involves intravenous injection of a radioactive isotope (usually technetium-99m pertechnetate). Uptake of the radioactive isotope is then assessed using a gamma camera to visualise functional salivary gland tissue.

Blood tests

These are carried out as there can be systemic involvement, which will become evident from the blood test results. The tests should include:

- Full blood count
- Erythrocyte sedimentation rate
- SS-A [Ro],
- SS-B [La],
- IgA immune complexes
- Rheumatoid factor

3   Answer any questions that they may have.

OSCE Station 6.6

A Differential diagnosis:

- Neoplastic and potentially malignant disease:
    - Leukoplakia
    - Carcinoma
    - Keratosis

- Inflammatory conditions:

    - Infective diseases: candidiasis, hairy leukoplakia, papilloma

- Non-infective conditions: lichen planus, lupus erythematosus

- Congenital:
    - White sponge naevus
    - Fordyce spots
    - Leukoedema

- Others:
    - Cheek-biting
    - Burns
    - Graft

B Diagnosis:

- History of presenting complaint

- Medical history:
    - Drugs – antibiotics, immunosuppressants, steroids may predispose to *Candida* infection
    - Underlying disease predisposing to *Candida* infection
    - Syphilis – rare cause of a white patch

- Dental history:
    - Restorations causing lichenoid reactions
    - Cheek-biting and trauma
    - Chemical burns

- Social history:
    - Possibility of high-risk group for keratosis, squamous-cell carcinoma

- Clinical examination:
  - Extra-oral – nodal involvement, associated angular cheilitis
  - Intra-oral

- Character of the patch:
  - Is it fixed or does it rub off (eg *Candida*)?
  - Is it uniform or is it striated – lichen planus, hairy leukoplakia, lupus?

- Site of patch:
  - Unilateral – idiopathic leukoplakia, squamous-cell carcinoma
  - Bilateral – lichen planus, Fordyce spots, white sponge naevus, cheek biting, *Candida*, submucous fibrosis
  - Localised or widespread
  - Sublingual – sublingual keratosis

- Local cause, eg friction from teeth

- Blood tests

- Swabs for *Candida*

- Incisional biopsy

- Answer any questions that the patient may have

OSCE Station 6.7

A Reticular lichen planus or lichenoid reaction.

B Clinical subtypes:

- Erosive/desquamative
- Papular
- Atrophic
- Plaque-like
- Bullous

C Predisposing factors:

- Drugs, eg antimalarials, antidiabetic drugs, non-steroidal anti-inflammatory drugs (NSAIDs), gold salts, antihypertensives
- Dental restorative materials, eg amalgam and gold
- Graft-versus-host disease
- Hepatitis C and chronic liver disease

D • Skin, nails and genitalia may be affected.

- Itchy, purple, raised patches are often seen on the wrists. They often occur following trauma – the Koebner phenomenon.
- If the skin of the scalp is affected, alopecia or hair loss may be seen.
- Nails appear ridged when affected.
- Genitalia show white lesions similar to those seen in the mouth.

OSCE Station 6.8

1   Introduce yourself politely to the patient.

2   Points to cover are given below.

Information

- Explain to the patient that this is a common condition called lichen planus.
- Some people have it on their skin, some in their mouth and others on their skin and in their mouth.
- It can last for many years.
- The cause is not known, but it can be set off by some drugs (eg antimalarials, antidiabetic drugs, NSAIDs) or dental restorative materials, eg amalgam.
- It is not infectious.

Management

- A biopsy, which involves taking a small sample of tissue, can give a definite diagnosis and exclude other causes.
- Blood tests can help exclude other conditions.
- If there are amalgam restorations adjacent to the lesions it may be advisable to have them replaced.
- If drugs are likely to be implicated, then it may be advisable to liaise with the patient's general medical practitioner to try alternatives.
- Regular monitoring is required to ensure that the disease does not progress.
- A subtype that affects the gingiva (gums) may make toothbrushing difficult.
- Spicy or salty food may make the lesions more sore.
- Treatment is aimed at alleviating the symptoms and may involve:
    - Benzydamine hydrochloride mouthwash (Difflam) to numb the sore area.
    - Topical steroids, eg betamethasone mouthwash, hydrocortisone (Corlan® pellets), triamcinolone acetonide.
    - If these do not provide relief then specialist care may be needed, which could involve steroids injected into the lesions themselves. In severe cases, steroids or steroid-sparing immunosuppressant

drugs may be needed systemically.
* Answer any questions that the patient may have.

OSCE Station 6.9

1   Introduce yourself politely to the patient.

2   Explain that the condition is common, affecting about 15% of the population.

3   Explain that the sores are caused by a virus called herpes simplex.

4   Explain that she would have been infected with the virus in the past, with or without symptoms. Although she recovered from the initial infection, the virus would have remained dormant in a nerve. The nerve involved is called the trigeminal nerve and it supplies the skin of the face and mouth area.

5   Explain that the virus is reactivated by various factors and causes cold sores. The activating factors include sunlight, menstruation, stress, fever, trauma and immunosuppression.

6   Reassure her that the lesions will normally come and go within 7–10 days.

7   Explain that the lesions are contagious so should not be touched.

8   Explain that treatment with antiviral agents (aciclovir) may help control the lesions, but must be used when the first symptoms of the lesions appear, ie when she feels any tingling or prickling. Aciclovir (Zovirax® cream 5%) should be applied five times a day to the lesion at the first sign of an attack.

9   Answer any questions that the patient may have.

OSCE Station 6.10

1 Introduce yourself politely to the patient.

2 Explain that you wish to gain her consent to remove a lump from her tongue.

Points to cover:

- The aim of the procedure is to remove the troublesome lump. If the lump is not removed, it may enlarge and will continue to be traumatised.
- Once removed, it should not recur unless that area is traumatised again.
- The procedure will be done under local anaesthesia, which means an injection or two to numb the area.
- Once it is numb, all they will feel is pressure, not pain. If they feel anything uncomfortable they should let the operator know and more local anaesthetic can be given.
- The lump will be removed and sent to the histopathology laboratory for examination under the microscope; this is routine practice for all lumps and bumps that are removed.
- The wound will be stitched with dissolving stitches but may bleed for a short while.
- Instructions on caring for the wound will be given after the procedure.
- The wound should heal in a week, but during that time the area will be a bit sore and swollen.
- Answer any questions that the patient may have.

3 Fill in the consent form and get the patient to read and sign it.

Comment

Different NHS trusts/primary care trusts have different policies on written consent. Some will not require a consent form to be filled in for a biopsy under local anaesthesia. The main purpose of gaining consent is to explain the procedure to the patient and ensure that they understand it and agree to have it carried out. This is more important than the actual signing of the form. However, to comply with local policy and to provide a written record it may be necessary to get the patient to sign a form. Getting a patient to sign a form without adequate explanation is *not* gaining consent.

OSCE Station 6.11

1 Place a suture through the lesion so that it can be held.

2 Make an elliptical incision around the base of the lesion. The incision should be no more than 0.5 cm deep to remove this polyp.

3 Remove the lesion by holding it by the suture.

4 Inform the examiner that you would put the lesion in a specimen pot with appropriate fixative and fill in the appropriate histopathology form.

5 Close the wound with interrupted sutures, to allow the edges to be nicely apposed.

6 Inform the examiner that you would apply pressure to the wound with gauze to achieve haemostasis and give the patient post-operative instructions.

b   **c**   **d**

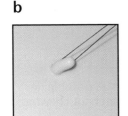 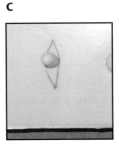 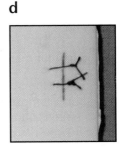

OSCE Station 6.12

1 Introduce yourself politely to the patient.

2 Explain to the patient that the biopsy showed some changes within the tissue, known as dysplasia, which literally translated means abnormal growth.

3 Explain that it is possible to get a whole spectrum of changes within tissue from completely normal at one end to carcinoma (cancer) at the other end. Between these two lie differing grades of dysplasia (mild, moderate and severe) and carcinoma in situ.
This biopsy showed mild dysplasia which means that there were some abnormalities within it but it is not carcinoma.

4 Explain that some lesions do progress to form carcinoma, however, some lesions regress. Reported rates for malignant change vary widely, so it is not possible to give an individual patient an exact rate. Having an area of dysplasia in the mouth means that the patient is at higher risk of getting lesions in other areas of the mouth and possibly of developing more than one carcinoma/cancer within their mouth.

5 Explain that management includes:

- Reducing as many predisposing factors as possible, ie, either smoking or chewing tobacco, betel nut chewing, high alcohol intake
- Treating any associated candidal infection if present
- Treating any underlying nutritional deficiencies

6 Explain that the patient may require long-term monitoring at regular intervals:

- If photographs have not been taken of the lesion(s) they should be done.
- There may be the need for repeat biopsies at later dates.
- Areas of mild dysplasia are not usually removed but if they progress then surgical removal is often carried out with cryotherapy, laser or by cutting it out.

7 Reassure the patient that they have not got oral cancer but that they need to be aware of the small potential of it developing.

8   Ask the patient if they have any questions.

CHAPTER 7
ORAL PATHOLOGY

Chapter 7: Questions

OSCE Station 7.1
5 minute station

Mrs Other has presented with a 6-week history of a painless swelling in the right buccal mucosa, as shown in the photograph below. She is otherwise fit and well. She is a non-smoker and consumes 8 units of alcohol a week.

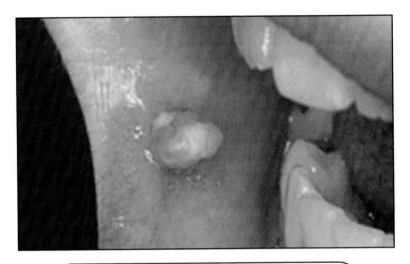

Mrs Ann Other

D.O.B 01.02.56

1232 Cromwell Road
Anytown
AB1 2CD

Hospital Number: 1234567XYZ

You decide to take an excisional biopsy of the lesion. With the help of the patient identification label, the clinical history and the photograph above, complete the pathology request form.

GENERAL DENTAL PRACTITIONER REQUEST FOR HISTOPATHOLOGICAL EXAMINATION BY POST

Please give patient details	Surname		Forename(s)		Ethnic origin (ring one): Asian Middle eastern Europe Mongoloid Negroid
	Date of Birth			Sex M / F	

Please give details of lesion	Differential diagnosis and clinical features:
	Medical History and **medications**:
	Smoking *type* *amount* *duration* **Alcohol** *type* *amount* *duration* **Betel qui**
	Also enclosed (please ring) Radiographs Clinical Pictures or Images e-mailed to: h&npath-dental@gstt.nhs

| Please mark extent of large lesions | |

Site of specimens or draw on diagram	Site 1 ring one: is this an incisional or excisional biopsy or curettage	Site 2 ring one: is this an incisional or excisional biopsy or curettage

Please give information for issuing report	Name of dentist and full practice address / practice stamp
	Posting information overleaf

	Date of biopsy	Report required by (date)

Residual sample is normally incinerated or used for quality assurance, NHS training, audit or research.
Please tick box if patient has indicated that they do NOT wish surplus tissue to be used for research ☐

OSCE Station 7.2
5 minute station

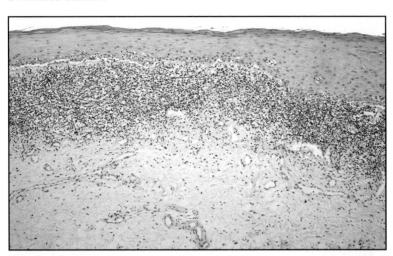

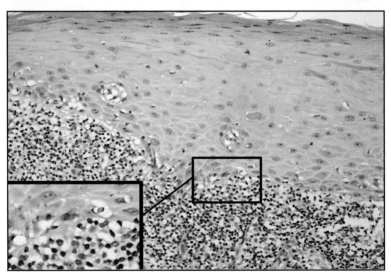

The photomicrograph above is from an incisional biopsy in a 50-year-old woman who presented with bilateral reticular white patches on the buccal mucosae. The reporting pathologist has stated that the features are consistent with lichen planus.

List the features that would have led the pathologist to arrive at this conclusion.

OSCE Station 7.3
5 minute station

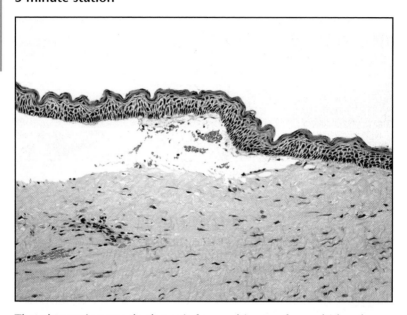

The photomicrograph above is from a biopsy of a multi-locular radiolucent lesion at the angle of the mandible.

A　Identify and label on the figure each of the following structures and features:

- Cyst wall
- Epithelial lining
- Erythrocytes
- Fibroblasts
- Surface corrugation
- Layer of parakeratinisation
- Basal palisading
- Separation of the epithelium from the corium

B　What is your diagnosis?

OSCE Station 7.4
5 minute station

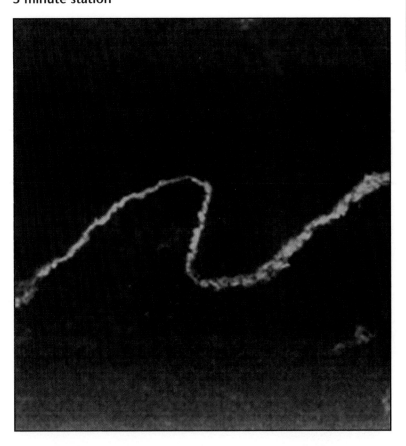

The illustration above shows a diagnostic test on a biopsy specimen of intra-oral blisters and ulcers.

A What is the diagnostic test?

B What special precautions do you need to consider when undertaking the biopsy?

C Please explain the stages involved in this test.

D What is your diagnosis?

OSCE Station 7.5
5 minute station

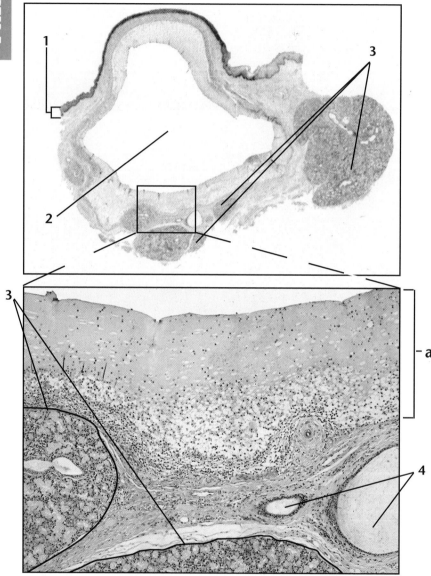

The photomicrographs shown above are from an excisional biopsy of a painless swelling of the lower lip.

A   Match the numbered labels with the following structures:

- Cyst lumen
- Surface epithelium
- Dilated salivary ducts
- Minor mucous glands

B   What is the predominant cell type in the area labelled 'a'?

C   What is your diagnosis and what treatment would you suggest for this patient?

OSCE Station 7.6
5 minute station

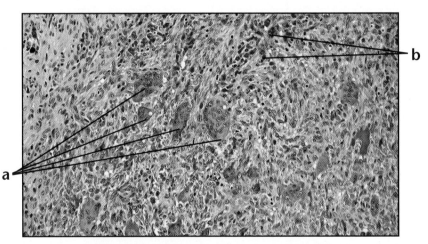

The photomicrograph above is from a biopsy of a well-defined unilocular radiolucency in the body of the mandible.

A   Name the cells labelled 'a'.

B   What is the likely cause of the pigmented area labelled 'b'?

C   Please give a differential diagnosis.

D   What other information is required to reach a definitive diagnosis?

OSCE Station 7.7
5 minute station

The following four photomicrographs are taken from a biopsy of a smooth red and white patch located on the dorsum of the tongue of a 67-year-old woman. a, b and c are haematoxylin and eosin stained sections at low, medium and high magnifications, respectively.

d is a high magnification photomicrograph of a special staining technique of the same field as c.

a

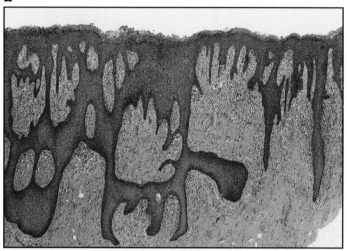

b

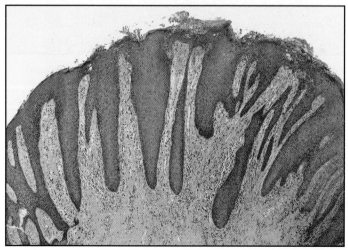

c

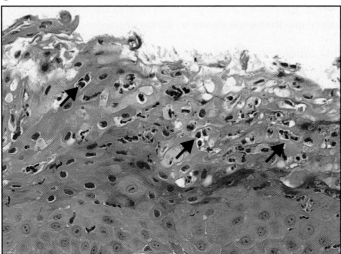

d

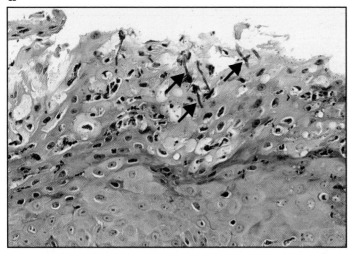

A Recalling the normal histological appearance of the dorsum of the tongue, what abnormal features are seen in figures a and b?

B c shows a thickened superficial spinous layer. What cells are the arrows pointing to?

C • What stain is used in figure d?
  • What structures are highlighted by the arrows?
  • Why are these not visible in figure c?

D What other intra-oral site does this condition commonly affect?

E What important possible sequelae of this condition do you need to consider when planning its management?

OSCE Station 7.8

A In the table below, place a tick in the box if the histological feature is indicative of epithelial dysplasia.

	Epithelial lymphocytosis		Increased number of nucleoli
	Nuclear pleomorphism		Apoptosis
	Basal mitoses		Loss of polarity of cells
	Increased nuclear: cytoplasmic ratio		Subepithelial hyalinisation
	Parakeratosis		Bulbous rete processes
	Premature keratinisation		Nuclear hyperchromatism
	Suprabasal mitoses		Koilocytosis
	Anisocytosis		Loss of cellular cohesion

Table 7.8a

B The following photomicrographs demonstrate epithelial dysplasia. Label the cytological features highlighted in parts a and b.

a

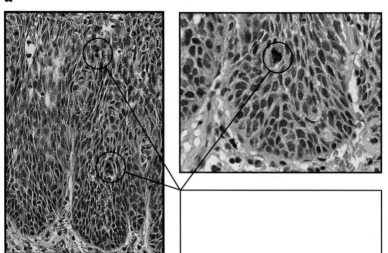

b

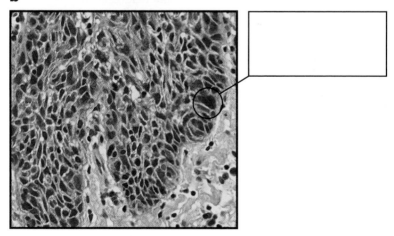

C How is oral epithelial dysplasia graded?

D What are the disadvantages of the current grading system of oral epithelial dysplasia?

Chapter 7: Answers

OSCE Station 7.1

The pathology request form is typical for any oral pathology unit. Points to note include:

- All writing must be legible.
- Patient and operator details need to be filled in fully.
- The specimen pot needs to be labelled.
- A brief clinical history needs to be provided, including:
  - Site
  - Size
  - Shape
  - Colour
  - Duration
  - Associated features
- It is important that the clinical differential diagnosis and clinical history are included. It cannot be assumed that a definitive diagnosis will be reached solely on histological grounds. The clinical differential diagnosis may be required to support the histological findings.
- In certain instances the radiographs or clinical photographs need to be submitted together with the biopsy specimen.
- It is important to summarise the medical history adequately. This is important as oral lesions may be a manifestation of systemic disease and/or drug reactions.
- A brief history of tobacco and alcohol consumption is also important.
- It must be indicated on the form whether the specimen is an incisional or an excisional biopsy. The pathologist may then be able to comment on the completeness of excision.

Comment

The marking scheme will be weighted so that the more important information, such as the clinical differential diagnosis, will be awarded a greater proportion of marks.

OSCE Station 7.2

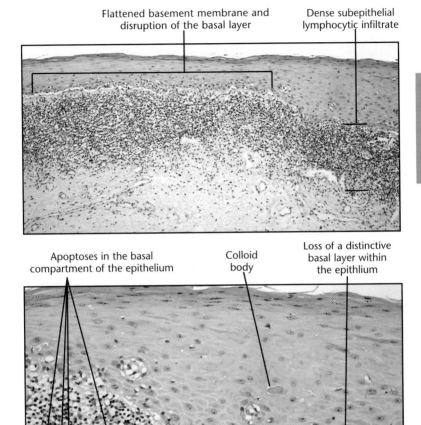

Flattened basement membrane and disruption of the basal layer

Dense subepithelial lymphocytic infiltrate

Apoptoses in the basal compartment of the epithelium

Colloid body

Loss of a distinctive basal layer within the epithlium

The pathologist would not have considered the histology in isolation, but would have taken into account the clinical history. In this case, the age and sex of the patient, together with the clinical distribution of the lesions, all support the histological diagnosis.

OSCE Station 7.3

A

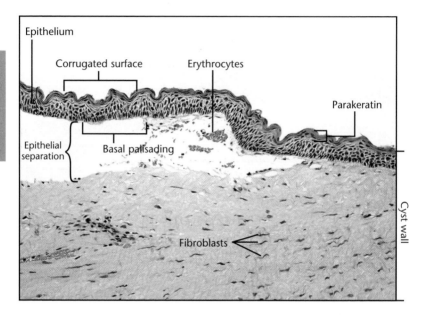

Epithelium

Corrugated surface

Erythrocytes

Parakeratin

Epithelial separation

Basal palisading

Fibroblasts

Cyst wall

B Taken together, the histological features are those of an odontogenic keratocyst. This is consistent with the clinical presentation as the majority of odontogenic keratocysts present as multilocular or pseudolocular radiolucencies, and the most frequent site is the angle of the mandible. Note that the cyst wall is not inflamed. Daughter or satellite cysts (not seen in this example) may also be present in the cyst wall. The presence of daughter cysts and the friable nature of the epithelial lining are considered to be reasons for the high rate of recurrence of these cysts.

OSCE Station 7.4

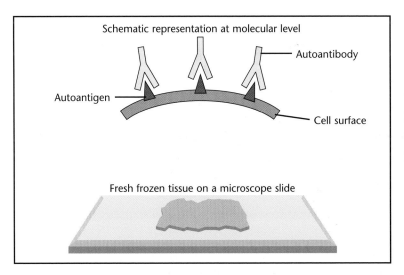

Schematic representation at molecular level

Autoantibody

Autoantigen

Cell surface

Fresh frozen tissue on a microscope slide

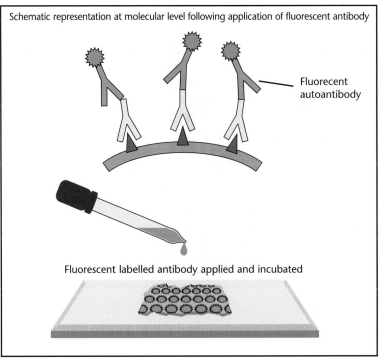

Schematic representation at molecular level following application of fluorescent antibody

Fluorecent autoantibody

Fluorescent labelled antibody applied and incubated

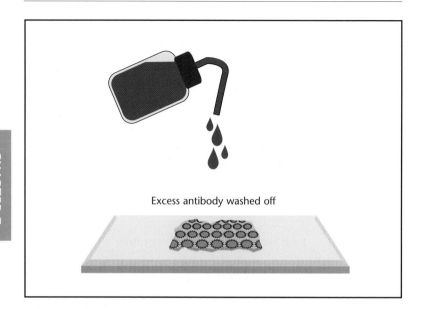

Excess antibody washed off

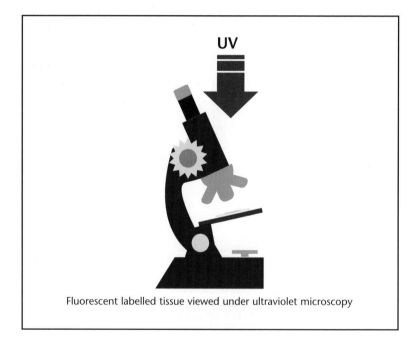

UV

Fluorescent labelled tissue viewed under ultraviolet microscopy

A   The test is direct immunofluorescence.

B   In immune-mediated vesiculobullous disorders, autoanti-bodies bind to antigenic sites, either on the epithelial cell surface or within the basement membrane zone, as in this example. The biopsy should be taken from para-lesional tissue as an intact epithelial–connective tissue interface is required. The tissue should be submitted fresh because formalin fixation destroys the antigenic sites.

C   The stages involved in direct immunofluorescence are as follows:

- Antibodies bound to a fluorescent marker are applied to the tissue section on the slide.
- These antibodies recognise the autoantibodies already bound in the tissue.
- The section is then washed and any bound fluorescent antibodies are viewed with a fluorescent microscope.
- The distribution of the fluorescent antibodies is equivalent to the distribution of the autoantibodies.

D   In this example, the antibody is distributed in a linear fashion along the basement membrane zone. Therefore, the likely diagnosis is mucous-membrane pemphigoid.

OSCE Station 7.5

A

1   Surface epithelium

2   Cyst lumen

3   Minor mucous glands

4   Dilated salivary ducts

B   In this example, the cyst lumen is not lined by epithelium and the predominant cell type at the periphery of the cyst is the foamy macrophage.

C   This is a mucus extravasation cyst (extravasation mucocoele). It is usually treated by excising the lesion and associated minor salivary gland. It could also be treated with cryotherapy.

OSCE Station 7.6

A   The cells labelled 'a' are osteoclast-like giant cells.

B   The pigment in the area labelled 'b' is haemosiderin. Note the prominent vascular stroma and the dense population of erythrocytes in the background.

C   This is giant-cell lesion and therefore the differential diagnosis will include:

- Central giant-cell granuloma
- Brown tumour of hyperparathyroidism
- Cherubism
- Aneurysmal bone cyst
- Other giant-cell lesions

D   To reach a definitive diagnosis, more information would be required, including:

- The age, sex and ethnic background of the patient
- The distribution of the lesion
- The radiological appearance
- Results of biochemical investigations

Comment

This OSCE highlights the necessity of considering the combination of clinical, radiological and histological features prior to reaching a definitive diagnosis.

OSCE Station 7.7

A   This is a case of chronic hyperplastic candidosis. The abnormality on low- and medium-power views is the loss of filiform papillae, which should be visible on normal dorsal lingual epithelium. This gives the clinical appearance of a smooth patch. A further abnormality consists of the elongated rete processes. These two features should raise the suspicion of candidosis even in low- and medium-magnification views.

B   The arrows are pointing to polymorphonuclear leucocytes (neutrophils) with typical multilobed nuclei. Neutrophil nuclei are about half the size of keratinocyte nuclei. Their presence in the superficial spinous layer together with irregular surface further raises the suspicion of candidal infection.

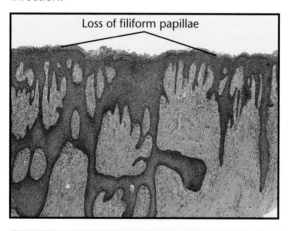

Loss of filiform papillae

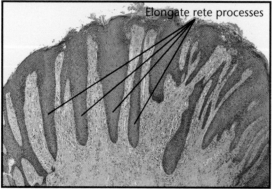

Elongate rete processes

C   The stain is periodic acid–Schiff (PAS), which stains glycogen, polysaccharides, mucin, mucoprotein, and glycoproteins magenta. The structures highlighted are fungal hyphae, whose walls are high in polysaccharides. These are not detected by standard haematoxylin and eosin staining.

D   Chronic hyperplastic candidosis affects the following oral sites in decreasing order of frequency: the buccal commissures, cheeks, palate and tongue.

E   Up to 15% of the chronic hyperplastic candidosis may progress to epithelial dysplasia. Furthermore, epithelial dysplasia associated with fungal infection significantly worsens over time in comparison with non-infected epithelial dysplasia. This underscores the importance of close monitoring of recalcitrant lesions that do not resolve after appropriate anti-fungal therapy.

OSCE Station 7.8

A

		✓	Increased number of nucleoli
	Epithelial lymphocytosis	✓	Increased number of nucleoli
✓	Nuclear pleomorphism		Apoptosis
	Basal mitoses	✓	Loss of polarity of cells
✓	Increased nuclear: cytoplasmic ratio		Subepithelial hyalinisation
	Parakeratosis	✓	Bulbous rete processes
✓	Premature keratinisation	✓	Nuclear hyperchromatism
✓	Suprabasal mitoses		Koilocytosis
✓	Anisocytosis	✓	Loss of cellular cohesion

Table 7.8b

B a: suprabasal mitoses; b: nuclear pleomorphism and hyperchromasia.

C Conventionally, epithelial dysplasia is graded as mild, moderate and severe. In general, the more prominent or numerous the above features, the more severe the grade of dysplasia. Another way is to divide the epithelium into thirds with the grades mild, moderate and severe dysplasia being assigned if the above features are limited to the inferior third, extend to the lower two-thirds or extend beyond the lower two-thirds of the epithelium, respectively.

D There is a considerable degree of subjectivity together with intra- and inter-observer variability. Furthermore, while severe dysplasia is more strongly associated with malignant transformation than mild or moderate dysplasia, grading of oral epithelial dysplasia remains an inconsistent prognostic indicator of progression to malignancy because squamous cell carcinomas can arise from mild or non-dysplastic epithelium.

DENTAL RADIOLOGY

Chapter 8: Questions

OSCE Station 8.1
5 minute station

This 16-year-old girl has a missing upper left canine. Radiographs are required to determine whether the tooth is impacted/unerupted.

Please seat the patient in the chair and set up the machine ready to take a radiograph of the appropriate area. (NB: you do not have access to a dental tomographic radiography machine.)

Props:

- Periapical films
- Occlusal films
- Film holders
- Cotton-wool rolls
- Gloves
- X-ray machine (not tomographic)

OSCE Station 8.2
5 minute station

When the radiograph of the 16-year-old girl with the missing left permanent canine in Station 8.1 is developed it is apparent that she has an unerupted permanent canine.

You need to determine the exact position of the tooth. What further radiographs could you take? Please set up the machine to take this view. When the radiograph is developed, how will you determine whether the tooth is buccally or lingually placed?

OSCE Station 8.3
5 minute station

The following radiographs have been taken by you in practice.

a **b** **c**

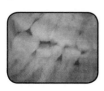 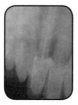 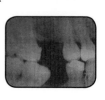

What is the problem with the images, why has it happened and how can it be avoided?

OSCE Station 8.4
5 minute station

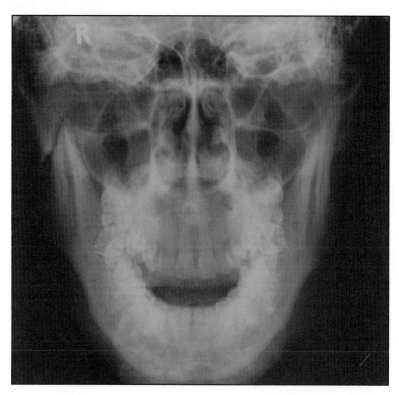

This is a radiograph taken of Mr John Smith, date of birth 14 February 1980, on 27 March 2005.

A   What radiographic view is this? How is it taken?

B   Please describe the radiograph.

OSCE Station 8.5
5 minute station

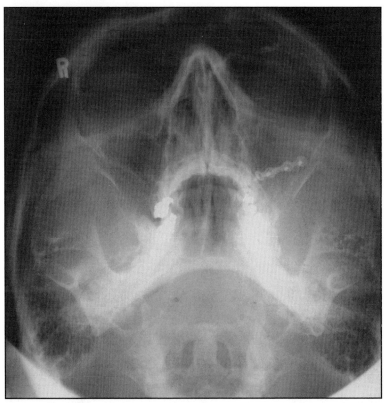

A   What radiographic view is this?

B   How would you go about describing it?

C   What interesting features can you see on this view?

OSCE Station 8.6
5 minute station

Please identify the labelled structures on the radiograph below.

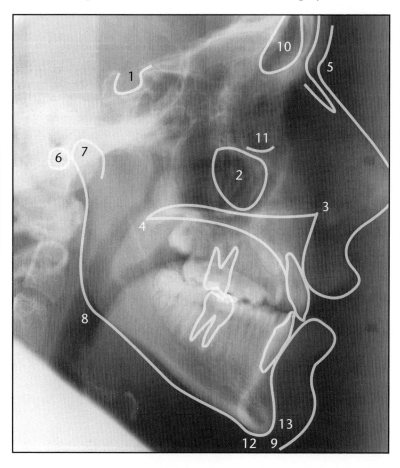

OSCE Station 8.7
5 minute station

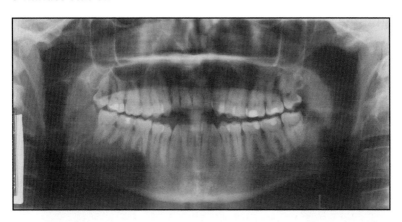

A What view is this?

B Please identify where you would expect to find the following structures on the radiograph:

1 Tongue shadow

2 Maxillary antrum

3 Coronoid process

4 Lingula

5 Mental foramen

6 Orbit

7 Styloid process

8 Ear lobe

9 Sigmoid notch

10 Nasolabial fold

OSCE Station 8.8
5 minute station

a

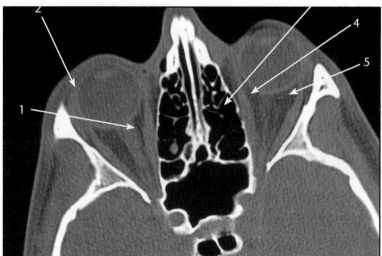

b

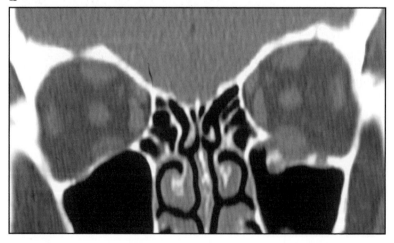

A   What planes are shown on these computed tomography (CT) scans?

B   Please identify the labelled structures and what abnormality is shown in CT scan b.

OSCE Station 8.9
5 minute station

You have been appointed radiation protection supervisor in your practice.

What are your responsibilities and what information must your written set of local rules include?

OSCE Station 8.10
5 minute station

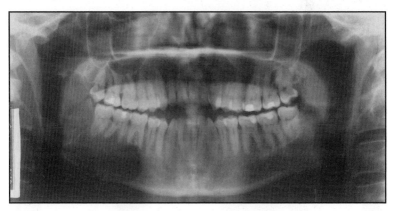

A What is this radiograph?

B How would you describe this lesion?

C What is the differential diagnosis?

OSCE Station 8.11
5 minute station

Look at the radiographs below and suggest the differential diagnosis for the appearance in each one.

a

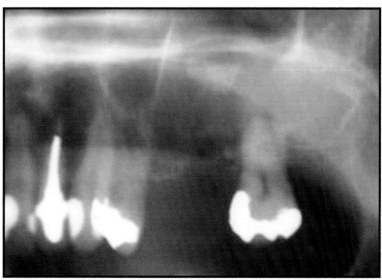

b

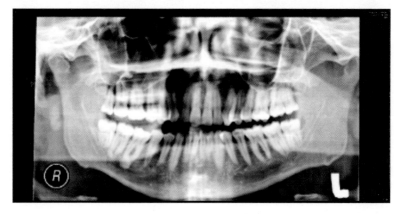

c

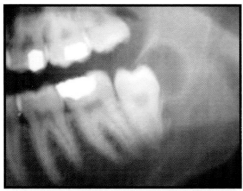

d

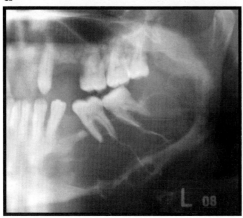

e

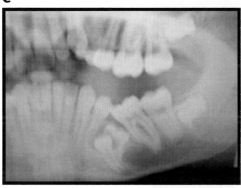

OSCE Station 8.12
5 minute station

Recommendations were made by NRPB/RCR in 1994 and targets set in 1998 to ensure the production of good diagnostic quality radiographs.

A   Describe the rating of radiographs.

B   Rate the following radiographs.

a

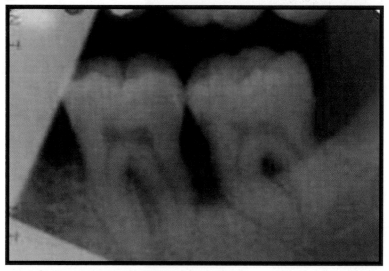

b

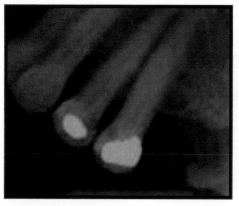

c

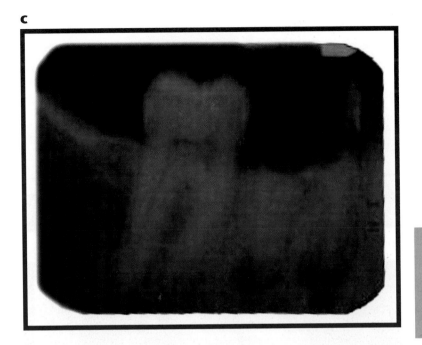

d

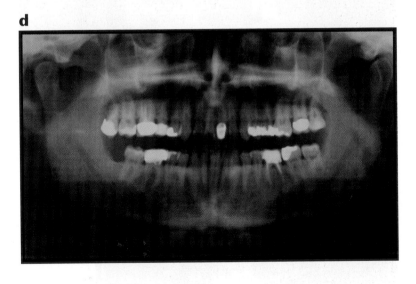

e

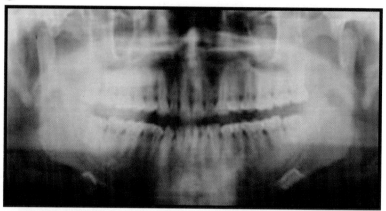

f

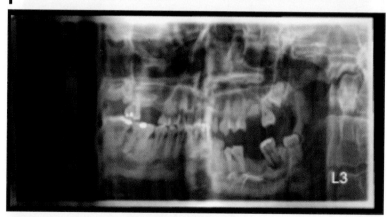

g

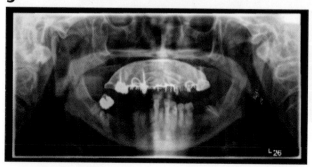

c   What are the minimum targets for radiographic quality?

Chapter 8: Answers

OSCE Station 8.1

Radiographs that could be taken include an upper periapical or an upper occlusal view.

Periapical view

There are two techniques for taking periapical radiographs, using either the paralleling method or the bisecting angle method. Explain to the patient that you are going to take a radiograph. (You would already have checked in her medical history that she is not pregnant.) Request her to remove her glasses and any orthodontic appliances (or dentures).

Paralleling technique

1   Place the file in a film holder to allow it to sit parallel to the tooth being X-rayed and aim the X-ray tube head at 90° to the film.

2   As the tooth in question is a maxillary canine, use an anterior film holder and a small film packet.

3   Place the film with the long axis parallel to the long axis of the tooth, with the smooth surface facing the tube head.

4   Position the patient comfortably on the chair with her head on the support. The patient is positioned with the occlusal plane horizontal.

5   Place the film in the patient's mouth with the film on the palatal side of the tooth and the film packet flat.

6   The patient bites gently on the film-holder to hold it in place.

7   Position the ring on the holder against the patient's skin.

8   Align the cone with the film holder ring.

9   Select the correct exposure for the machine in question.

Bisecting angle technique

1   Position the patient as for the paralleling technique.

2   Place the film on the palatal aspect of the tooth in question using either the patient's finger to hold it or a film holder (± cotton-wool rolls). The long axis of the film should be as close as possible to the tooth whilst keeping the film flat.

3   Angle the tube at 50° to the horizontal so that the beam is at 90° to the angle between the tooth and the film packet. The beam must be positioned in the vertical plane to allow the whole of the tooth to be visualised on the film.

4   Select the correct exposure for the machine.

Upper standard occlusal view

1   Position the patient as for the paralleling technique.

2   Give the patient a thyroid shield to hold under her chin.

3   The film is held in place in the patient's mouth by the patient biting gently against it so that it lies against the occlusal surfaces of the upper anterior teeth.

4   Angle the tube downwards at 65–70° to the horizontal to aim through the bridge of the nose.

5   Select the correct exposure for the machine.

OSCE Station 8.2

The parallax technique can be used to determine the exact position of teeth. It works on the principle that when two radiographs are taken those objects further away from the tube move in the same direction as the tube and those closer to the tube move in the opposite direction. It is often remembered by the acronym 'SLOB' – same lingual, opposite buccal. When a tooth lies in the line of the arch it will not move with a shift in tube position. The parallax technique can be performed in a horizontal plane with:

- two periapical views, and
- two occlusal views;

or it can be performed in the vertical plane with

- an occlusal and a periapical
- a panoramic radiograph and a periapical or occlusal.

In this instance no panoramic facilities are available, so occlusals and periapicals can be used. If a periapical was taken in Station 8.1, then another periapical can be taken by the same method, but the tube will need to be shifted. It is most commonly shifted in the horizontal plane. So if the tube was centred over the canine in the first view it can be centred over the lateral or central incisor in the second view. Hence the patient and film should be positioned as before and the tube moved horizontally (see Station 8.1).

If an occlusal radiograph was taken previously, then a periapical can now be taken using the parallelling technique. This will enable vertical parallax to be carried out. The patient should be positioned as in Station 8.1 and a periapical taken. Alternatively, another occlusal view can now be taken to enable horizontal parallax to be carried out. The patient should be positioned as for an upper standard occlusal view in Station 8.1. The film is then centred on the side of the mouth under investigation, and the patient bites gently on it to hold it in place. The tube should be angled downwards at 65–70° to the horizontal and centred on the cheek. This will provide enough horizontal tube shift to allow horizontal parallax to be carried out.

Comment

Several other methods are available for localisation of unerupted teeth:

- A vertex occlusal
- A true lateral and postero-anterior view of the jaws (two views at right angles)
- Stereoscopic views
- Cross-sectional spiral tomography

OSCE Station 8.3

Image a

Bite wings showing severe overlap of contact points, required teeth not shown (premolars).

Cause – Film placed too far back in the mouth; horizontal angle greater or less than 90°.

To avoid – Ensure film is parallel to teeth, mesial surface against lower canine; align beam at 90° to arch.

Image b

Lower canine periapical, teeth all elongated and missing apices.

Cause – Too shallow a beam.

To avoid – Correct use of bisecting angle, increase the occlusal plane/tube-head angle; correct use of film holder.

Image c

Image too dark.

Cause – Overexposure.

To avoid – Check exposure is correct.

OSCE Station 8.4

A This is a postero-anterior view of the mandible (PA mandible). It is taken by positioning the patient so that the line from the outer canthus of the eye to the external auditory meatus is horizontal, and their forehead and tip of the nose touch the film. The tube head is positioned horizontally. The beam is centred on the cervical spine so as to pass between the rami of the mandible.

B This is a postero-anterior view of the mandible (PA mandible) taken on 27 March 2005 of Mr John Smith aged, 25, a fully dentate patient. It shows the whole of the mandible and the mid-face. Clearly visible is a displaced fracture of the right mandibular condyle with significant shortening of ramus height. The fractured segment is minimally angulated. Another fracture is visible in the right parasymphyseal region.

OSCE Station 8.5

A   This is a 30° occipito-mental (OM) radiograph.

B   The best way of describing radiographs is a systematic approach. The approach for OM views commonly used is based on that suggested by McGrigor and Campbell, hence the name 'Campbell's lines'.

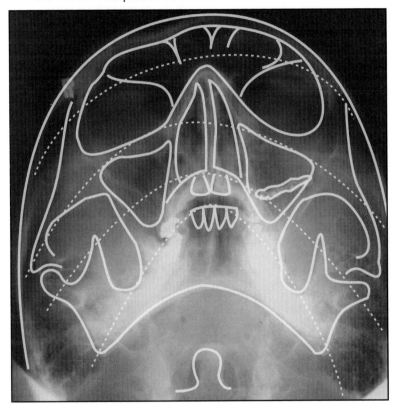

- The system follows four curves or lines across the film, from one side to the other.
- The most inferior line goes from one angle of mandible through the occlusal plane to the other angle of the mandible.
- The next line goes from the neck of the condyle on one side up through the coronoid process, on through the lateral wall of the maxillary antrum, through the base of

the nose, and back down through the other lateral wall of the maxillary antrum and so on to the other condyle.
- The next line goes from the zygomatic arch on one side, through the body of the zygoma, through the infra-orbital rim and through the nasal complex, then back down the other side through the infra-orbital rim and on to the zygomatic arch.
- The most superior line goes from the fronto-zygomatic suture on one side, through the supra-orbital ridge, through the frontal sinus and then down the other side though the same structures.

Once these have been examined and any abnormalities noted, then other anatomical outlines are examined on both sides, including:

- Lateral walls of the nose
- Orbital rims
- Edges of the temporal bones extending along the zygomatic arches
- Zygomatic

C This radiograph shows evidence of a previous fractured left zygoma. The fracture has been reduced but there is still a step visible in the lateral wall of the left maxillary antrum. There are no steps visible in the fronto-zygomatic region or the zygomatico-temporal region. There is a mini bone plate present on the left anterior maxillary wall. The maxillary antra are clear with no evidence of a fluid level.

OSCE Station 8.6

1 Sella turcica

2 Maxillary antrum

3 Anterior nasal spine

4 Posterior nasal spine

5 Nasion

6 External auditory meatus

7 Condyle

8 Gonion

9 Gnathion

10 Frontal sinus

11 Infra-orbital rim

12 Menton

13 Pogonion

OSCE Station 8.7

A This is a dental panoramic tomograph.

B

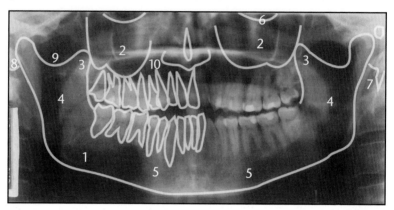

OSCE Station 8.8

When describing radiographs or scans it is usual to mention the patient's name and the date the radiographs were taken, eg: 'These are computed tomographic scans (CT) of the orbits of Mr X, taken on …… (date).'

a

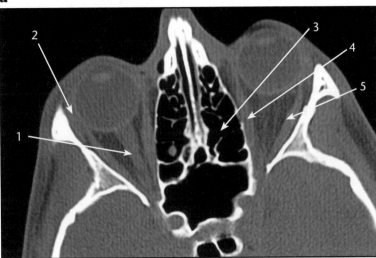

b

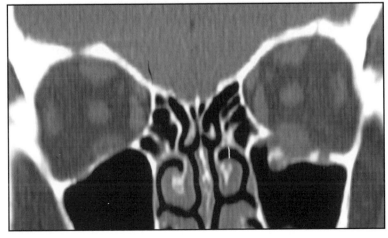

A

(a) Axial CT to show orbits

(b) Coronal CT to show herniating tissue into antrum

B

Structures labelled on CT scan a:

1   Optic nerve

2   Lacrimal gland

3   Ethmoid sinus

4   Medial rectus muscle

5   Lateral rectus muscle

CT scan b is a coronal section of CT which shows herniating tissue into the antrum associated with a left orbital floor fracture. Clinical signs associated with an orbital floor fracture:

- Double vision (diplopia)
- Limitation of eye movement (ophthalmoplegia)
- Lowered pupillary level on affected side (hypoglobus)
- Sunken eye (enophthalmos)
- Numbness/tingling of cheek (paraesthesia, anaesthesia of infraorbital nerve)

OSCE Station 8.9

Responsibilities

- The radiation protection supervisor (RPS) can be either a dentist or a senior member of staff in the dental practice.
- The RPS must be adequately trained and have sufficient authority to implement their responsibilities.
- The RPS is appointed to comply with the Ionising Radiation Regulations 1999 (IRR99).

Information included in 'Local Rules'

The 'Local Rules' relating to radiation protection must be written, and they must include certain information:

- Your name as the radiation protection supervisor.
- The 'controlled area', (1.5 m around the X-ray tube and patient and anywhere in the path of the primary beam until it is attenuated by either a solid wall or distance) must be identified and described.
- Names of staff qualified to take radiographs.
- Details of their training.
- Working instructions.
- What to do in the event of equipment malfunction.
- What to do in the event of accidental exposure to radiation.
- Name of the person who has legal responsibility to ensure compliance with the regulations.
- Details and results of dose investigation levels.
- Name and contact details of the radiation protection Advisor (RPA).
- Arrangements for personal dosimetry.
- Arrangements for pregnant staff.
- Reminder to staff of their legal responsibilities under IRR99.

OSCE Station 8.10

A   This is a dental panoramic tomogram (DPT).

B   When describing a lesion on a radiograph it is usual to cover the following points:

- Radiodensity
- Site
- Size
- Shape
- Outline
- Adjacent structures

With regard to this lesion there is a radiolucent lesion at the angle of the mandible on the right hand side, extending from the apex of the lower second premolar right up to the sigmoid notch area. It is multilocular and has a well-corticated margin. It has not resorbed the roots of the adjacent teeth and it is not possible to evaluate its relation to the inferior dental nerve. The lesion is not a normal anatomical structure and is not due to an artefact, hence it is likely to be pathological.

C   Common radiolucent lesions in the mandible include:

- Cysts
- Tumours
- Giant-cell lesions
- Infections
- Traumatic lesions
- Idiopathic lesions

Common multilocular radiolucent lesions in the mandible include:

- Cysts – keratocysts
- Odontogenic tumours – ameloblastoma, Pindborg's tumour (calcifying epithelial odontogenic tumour), odontogenic fibroma, odontogenic myxoma
- Central giant cell-lesions

A definitive diagnosis is only possible after a biopsy.

OSCE Station 8.11

When answering a question regarding likely radiological diagnosis and its differential diagnosis, it is important to take account of the following:

- Site or anatomical position of the lesion
- Size of the lesion
- Shape of the lesion
- Outline/edge or periphery of the lesion
- Relative radiodensity
- Effect on adjacent structures.

The above information will elicit a list of possible diagnoses although the final diagnosis may require histological confirmation.

a
- Site: maxillary antrum
- Size: small
- Shape: conical
- Relative radiodensity: radiopaque (same density as root)
- Effect on adjacent structures: discontinuity of antral floor.

The likely diagnosis is a displaced root in the maxillary antrum with evidence of an oroantral communication.

b
- Site: apex of lower right first molar
- Size: 1 cm
- Shape: round lesion appears attached to root
- Outline: well defined
- Relative radiodensity: radio-opaque (may be surrounded by a thin radiolucent line – but not obvious in this image)
- Effect on adjacent structures: attached to root, which is obscured

The likely diagnosis for a well-defined radio-opaque lesion at apex of the lower right first molar is benign cementoblastoma (true cementoma). The differential diagnosis is cemental dysplasia – usually lower incisor teeth, radiolucent in early stage but radio-opaque in late stage.

c
- Site: associated with crown of lower left third molar
- Size: 1 cm
- Shape: round, monolocular
- Outline: smooth, well corticated

- Relative radiodensity: uniformly radiolucent
- Effect on adjacent structures: associated with an unerupted tooth.

This radiographs shows pericoronal lesion which is likely to be a dentigerous cyst.

Differential diagnosis:

- Normal follicular space (suspect cyst if the follicular space is greater than 3 mm)

d
- Site: body/angle of the mandible extending into ramus
- Size: large (in this case – from the premolars to almost the sigmoid notch)
- Shape: multi-locular (can be mono-locular)
- Outline: smooth, well defined and corticated
- Relative radiodensity: radiolucent with internal radio-opaque septa
- Effect on adjacent structures: minimal displacement of adjacent tooth, no resorption, not seen in this image but usually causes displaced, loosened and resorbed teeth with extensive expansion in all dimensions. Most likely diagnosis of this multi-locular radiolucency extending from the body to the ascending ramus of the mandible with evidence of expansion of the lower border is ameloblastoma.

Differential diagnosis:

- Keratocyst: same site, pesudo-locular or multi-locular, uniformly radiolucent, minimal displacement of adjacent tooth, rarely have resorbed roots.
- Myxoma: posterior mandible or maxilla. Young adults, can be mono- or multi-locular. Radiolucent with fine septa ('strings of tennis racket'), bone expansion, loose or displaced teeth.
- Aneurysmal bone cyst: adolescence, same site, mono- or multi-locular, soap bubble appearance, teeth displaced but rarely show resorption.
- Central haemangioma.
- Giant cell granuloma.
- Cherubism: consider this as a differential diagnosis if the same appearance is seen in a child 2–6 years of age,with displacement of deciduous teeth and extensive expansion. It can present in maxilla.

e Crowded dentition with a infra-occluded lower left primary second molar and impacted lower left second premolar.

OSCE Station 8.12

A Rating of radiographs

Rating	Quality	Basis
1	Excellent	No errors of exposure, positioning or processing
2	Diagnostically acceptable	Some errors of exposure, positioning or processing, but which do not detract from the diagnostic utility of the radiograph
3	Unacceptable	Errors of exposure, positioning or processing which render the radiograph unacceptable

Table 8.12a

B
- (a) Rating 2 – Coning
- (b) Rating 3 – Apical tissue not seen
- (c) Rating 1 – No errors of exposure, positioning or processing
- (d) Rating 1 – No errors of exposure, positioning or processing
- (e) Rating 2 – Overexposed, but still able to use diagnostically
- (f) Rating 3 – Errors of positioning (patient moved), rendering the radiograph unacceptable
- (g) Rating 3 – Patient has upper denture in situ, which rendered the radiograph unacceptable

C The minimum targets for radiographic quality

Rating	Percentage of radiographs taken
1	Not less than 70%
2	Not greater than 20%
3	Not greater than 10%

Table 8.12b

HUMAN DISEASE INCLUDING EMERGENCIES

Chapter 9: Questions

OSCE Station 9.1
5 minute station

You are a dentist in general practice and a patient who has just walked into your surgery collapses. Describe how you would proceed.

OSCE Station 9.2
5 minute station

You are a dentist in general practice. You are about to start treatment on a patient when they complain of feeling unwell and start fitting. Describe how you will proceed.

OSCE Station 9.3
5 minute station

You are a dentist in general practice. You have just given a patient a local anaesthetic and she suddenly becomes short of breath and develops swelling of her lips. Describe how you would proceed, using a mannequin.

OSCE Station 9.4
5 minute station

You are an SHO and need to take a blood sample for a full blood count from a patient attending for an assessment prior to surgery. Please obtain a sample from the mannequin's arm and explain your actions as you proceed.

Props:

- Mannequin arm
- Tourniquet
- Sterile wipe

- Needle
- Vacutainer®
- Blood tube
- Gloves
- Cotton-wool rolls
- Adhesive plaster
- Sharps bin

OSCE Station 9.5
5 minute station

The pulse and blood pressure of this 68-year-old man needs to be recorded. Please show how you will do this.

Props:

- Stethoscope
- Sphygmomanometer
- Mannequin arm or patient

OSCE Station 9.6
5 minute station

You are fitting a posterior crown, and the crown slips from your fingers and disappears. The patient coughs and becomes distressed.

A What signs are suggestive of airway obstruction?

B What action would you take?

OSCE Station 9.7
5 minute station

A Identify the equipment shown and what are the devices used for?

a

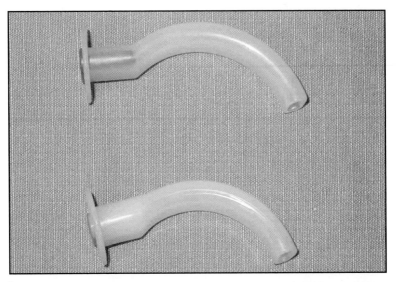

b

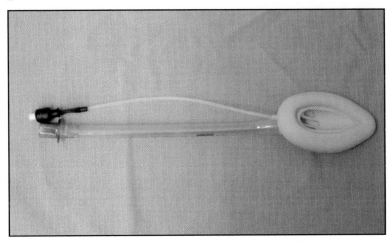

c

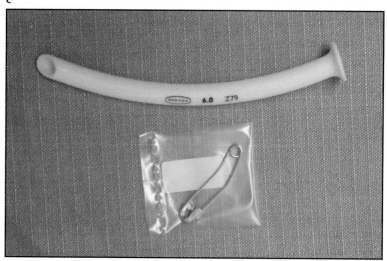

d

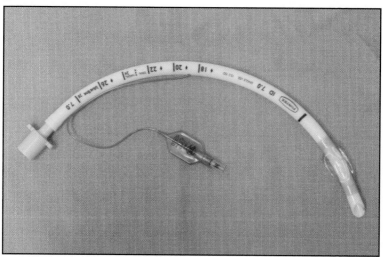

B With regard to device (a), how would you decide which size of device to use for a patient and how is it inserted?

C With regard to device (c), how would you decide which size of device to use for a patient?

OSCE Station 9.8
5 minute station

A Please work out the BMI of these three patients. Based on the BMI alone would any of these patients not be suitable for intravenous sedation in a dental practice?

Patient	Height	Weight
A	1 m 53 cm	50 kg
B	1 m 88 cm	98 kg
C	1 m 75 cm	74 kg

Table 9.8a

B At what BMI would a patient be categorised as being obese?

C Here is the ASA grading for patients requiring general anaesthesia.

Grade	Description
Grade 1	Healthy patient
Grade 2	A patient with a disease causing mild to moderate systemic disturbance
Grade 3	A patient with a disease causing severe systemic disturbance
Grade 4	A patient with a life-threatening disease
Grade 5	A moribund patient with little chance of survival with or without surgery

Table 9.8b

Please allocate the following patients to the correct ASA grade.
1   A patient with treated anti-hypertensive drugs who is now stable
2   A patient with chronic obstructive airway disease
3   A patient with unstable angina
4   A patient with stable diabetes mellitus

OSCE Station 9.9
15 minute station

A patient attends your dental surgery with the following medical history and require extraction of a lower second molar. What further information do you need to obtain from them? Explain to them what the concerns are with respect to them having a dental extraction and what additional measures you would take.
History:

A   Taking bisphosphonates
B   Taking warfarin for atrial fibrillation
C   Has diabetes mellitus

Chapter 9: Answers

OSCE Station 9.1

1   Check the area for danger.

2   Assess the patient and see if they respond. If there is no response, follow the algorithm of basic life support commonly remembered as 'ABC': **Airway/Breathing/Circulation**. If they are breathing and they have a pulse it is most likely that they have fainted.

Fainting

This presents with dizziness, nausea, pallor, feeling cold and clammy, and a slow thready pulse.

1   Place the victim in the supine position, elevate legs/position head below the level of the heart.

2   Loosen clothing.

3   Monitor the pulse.

4   Determine the cause and avoid in the future.

5   If recovery is slow, reconsider the cause.

Adult Basic Life Support

The flowchart overleaf shows a basic life support algorithm.

Continue resuscitation until help arrives and the care of the patient is taken over or until the victim shows signs of life.

Please check the Resuscitation Council UK guidelines for updates www.resus.org.uk

Check for danger

↓

Check for responsiveness by shaking and shouting

↓

No response

↓

Shout for help

↓

Open airway by head tilt/chin lift and manual clearance of mouth

↓

Check breathing: **look** (chest movement), **listen** (breath sounds), **feel** (breath on cheek) for no more than 10 seconds

↓   ↓

No breathing

If breathing present, place the patient in recovery position, then go for help

↓

Go for help – call ambulance

↓

Cardiopulmonary resuscitation: 30 chest compressions followed by two breaths. Rate of 100 chest compressions/minute

OSCE Station 9.2

1 Stop what you are doing.

2 Remove all items from the patient's mouth.

3 Establish their symptoms? Aura: flashing lights, *déjà vu*, familiar smell/sensation.

4 Recheck their medical history if time permits.

5 Call for help.

6 When fitting commences, place in the recovery position if possible. If not possible, leave the patient in the dental chair but remove any equipment from the area so they do not injure themselves on it.

7 Maintain the airway.

8 Give oxygen via a mask.

9 Check the pulse, oxygen saturation if available (pulse oximeter).

10 Establish intravenous access.

11 If the patient recovers, monitor and arrange for them to be seen by their general practitioner if they are known to be epileptic: or send the patient to hospital.

12 If there is repeat fitting (status epilepticus), or patient not recovering, give intravenous diazepam (5–10 mg over 2 minutes). If IV accession is not available rectal diazepan can be used.

13 Assess for respiratory depression.

14 Call for an ambulance.

OSCE Station 9.3

1   Stop what you are doing.

2   Call for help.

3   Put the patient in a position of comfort. Lying flat, with or without leg elevation may be helpful for hypotension, but it is unhelpful for patients with breathing difficulties.

4   Give oxygen via a mask, 10–15 L/minute.

5   Give 0.5 mL 1:1000 (500 micrograms epinephrine [adrenaline]) intramuscularly. This should be repeated after 5 minutes unless the patient improves. In some cases several doses may be needed. NB: If adults are treated with an EpiPen® remember that it only contain 300 micrograms, which will usually be sufficient, but may need to be repeated. Intravenous adrenaline is hazardous and is only used in patients with profound shock and by those experienced in its use and with cardiac monitoring.

6   Establish intravenous access.

7   Give 10–20 mg chlorphenamine (an H_1-antihistaminic) by slow intravenous injection or intramuscularly if intravenous route is unavailable. Hydrocortisone (as sodium succinate) 100–500 mg intramuscularly or slowly intravenously should be administered after severe attacks to help prevent late sequelae – this is especially important in asthmatic patients. An inhaled β_2 agonist such as salbutamol may be a useful adjunct. An H_2 blocker should be considered.

8   If severe hypotension does not respond to drug treatment then a rapid infusion of 1–2 L of fluid may be needed.

NB: If the patient proceeds to cardiac arrest, cardiopulmonary resuscitation must be performed (see Station 9.1).

Comment

Differential diagnosis:

  • Acute asthma

- Angio-oedema
- Other drug interaction/reaction, eg intravascular injection of local anaesthetic

OSCE Station 9.4

1 Introduce yourself politely to the patient.

2 Check the patient's identity.

3 Explain the procedure in a clear and succinct manner and gain consent to proceed.

4 Check that the correct equipment is available before starting the procedure.

5 Put on the gloves.

6 Place the tourniquet on the arm.

7 Select an appropriate vein.

8 Clean the skin with an alcohol wipe.

9 Connect the needle with the Vacutainer® correctly.

10 Warn the patient that they will feel a sharp scratch.

11 Insert the needle at approximately 35–45°.

12 Connect the blood tube with the end of the Vacutainer.®

13 Remove the blood tube when there is an adequate amount of blood in it.

14 Release the tourniquet.

15 Remove the Vacutainer® and the needle.

16 Cover the puncture wound with cotton wool/alcohol wipe and ask the patient to press on the area.

17 Place a plaster over the wound after ascertaining that the patient is not allergic to plasters.

18 Dispose of sharps appropriately.

19 Tell the examiner that you would label the tube and fill in the appropriate form.

Do everything in as clean and fluent a manner as possible.

OSCE Station 9.5

1 Introduce yourself politely to the patient.

2 Check the patient's identity.

3 Explain that you wish to take their pulse and gain their permission.

4 Check the radial artery pulse and calculate the beats per minute.

5 Explain the blood pressure procedure, stating that a cuff will be wrapped around the patient's arm, which will be tightened and may feel a bit uncomfortable.

6 Obtain their permission to proceed.

7 Select an appropriately-sized cuff.

8 Attach the equipment and check that it is working.

9 Wrap the cuff around the arm: the bladder should lie over the brachial artery, and the patient's arm should be level with his heart.

10 Increase the pressure while palpating the brachial or radial artery. When the pulse disappears note the systolic pressure. (palpatory method).

11 Allow the cuff to fully deflate and then re-inflate it to at least 20 mmHg over the reading you just noted by the palpatory method, with the stethoscope over the brachial artery.

12 Deflate the cuff slowly, listening and watching the gauge. The point at which the sounds appear indicate the systolic pressure (Korotkoff I).

13 Continue to deflate slowly until the sounds disappear, indicating the diastolic pressure (Korotkoff V).

14 Deflate the cuff.

The entire procedure should be done in a fluent manner. To rule out postural hypotension it would be necessary to repeat the procedure but with the patient lying down and standing up.

OSCE Station 9.6

Points to cover are given below.

Signs of airway obstruction

- A conscious patient with airway obstruction will complain of difficulty in breathing, may be choking and will be distressed.
- Airway obstruction can be partial or total.
- Partial airway obstruction results in noisy breathing.
- In complete airway obstruction there is no noise as there is no air movement.
- If respiratory movements are present they will be strenuous and the accessory muscle of respiration will be used.
- There will be see-saw movements of the chest and abdomen, with the chest being drawn in on inspiration and the abdomen being drawn in on expiration.

Management

1 If airway blockage is only partial the patient will usually be able to dislodge the foreign body by coughing:

- So while the patient is conscious and breathing despite evidence of obstruction you should encourage them to continue coughing.
- Sit the chair upright.

2 If the obstruction is complete or the patient becomes exhausted or cyanosed, then you should carry out back slaps:

- Remove any other debris from the patient's mouth.
- Sit the patient upright and support their chest with one hand while leaning them well forwards.
- Give five sharp slaps to their back in-between their scapulae with the heel of your hand. If the obstruction is relieved it may not be necessary to give all five slaps.

3 If the slaps fail, carry out abdominal thrusts.

- These are best carried out by standing behind the patient, but the patient can be seated or standing.
- Bend the patient forwards.
- Place both your arms round the upper part of their abdomen.

- Clench your fist and place it between the umbilicus and the bottom end of the sternum.
- Grasp the fist with your other hand.
- Pull sharply upwards and inwards. This should dislodge the obstructing object.
- If it is not dislodged, recheck the mouth for any obstruction that can be reached with a finger.
- Continue alternating five back slaps with five abdominal thrusts.

4   If the patient becomes unconscious, the associated muscle relaxation may allow air to pass into the lungs. You then need to carry out the sequence of basic life support (as in Station 9.1).

OSCE Station 9.7

A   They are all airway adjuncts:

a = Guedal airway
b = Laryngeal mask airway (LMA)
c = nasopharyngeal airway
d = Endotracheal tube

B   A Guedel or oropharyngeal airway is a curved plastic tube (a) with a flange at the oral end. It is flattened to allow it to fit between the tongue and the hard palate. To estimate the size, the airway should be as long as the vertical distance from the angle of the mandible to the mandibular incisors.

Insertion

- Care must be taken to prevent the tongue from being pushed back on insertion.
- The mouth is opened and checked for debris as this may be pushed into the larynx when inserting the airway.
- The airway is inserted with the opening facing the hard palate, ie in an upside-down manner, until the end is at the junction of the hard and soft palate.
- The airway is rotated 180° so that its curve follows the curve of the tongue.
- It is then advanced until it lies in the oropharynx.
- If the patient gags or strains the device should be removed; they are suitable only for unconscious patients.
- Once the device is seated in place the airway should be opened by a head tilt or chin lift.
- The patency of the airway and ventilation should be checked by the 'look, listen and feel' technique.

C   The nasopharyngeal airway (c) is a soft tube with a flange at one end and a bevel at the other. This is sized in millimetres according to the internal diameter of the tube, with sizes 6 and 7 usually being used for adults. It is said that the tube used should have the same diameter as the patient's little finger. It is better tolerated in patients who are not deeply unconscious.

The laryngeal mask airway or LMA (b) consists of a wide-bore tube with an elliptical cuff that is designed to make a seal around the laryngeal opening. The endotracheal tube (d) provides a secure airway, as the tube passes through the larynx and into the trachea.

OSCE Station 9.8

A • BMI is a calculation used to estimate the proportion of body weight that fat accounts for.
• To work it out the patient's weight in kilograms is divided by the square of their height in metres, ie BMI = weight (kg)/height (m) x height (m)

Patient	BMI
A	21.4
B	27.8
C	24.2

Table 9.8c

B Patients A and C are in the ideal range and patient B is overweight but based on this alone there is no contraindication to sedation in the dental practice.

Description	Value
Underweight	<18
Ideal	18–25
Overweight	>25
Obese	>30

Table 9.8d

NB These ranges should be slightly increased for the elderly and for females.

C 1 A treated hypertensive patient – ASA grade 2

2 A patient with chronic obstructive airway disease – ASA grade 3

3 A patient with unstable angina – ASA grade 4

4 A patient with stable diabetes mellitus – ASA grade 2

OSCE Station 9.9

It is important to take a thorough medical history from all patients. For patients with a medical condition that may influence/ affect their dental treatment it is necessary to find out all necessary information and take steps to minimise any adverse outcome.

1 Introduce yourself politely to the patient.

2 Patient complaint – Find out whether they need the extraction to be carried out or whether there is an alternative treatment option.

NB: With these patients primary prevention of disease is best.

A Bisphosphonates

1 Explain to the patient that as they are on bisphosphonates they are at risk of impaired healing of the bone after the extraction (bisphosphonates-related osteonecrosis of the jaw: (BRONJ). The risk depends on a number of factors:
   - Are they on an oral or intravenous agent (osteoporosis usually oral [occasionally IV] or malignancy often intravenous)?
   - How long have they been taking the agent?

2 If the patient is taking oral bisphosphonates (which is likely to be a large proportion of patients seen in dental practice), reassure them that the risk is very low.

3 Check if they have other concurrent risk factors for BRONJ, eg diabetes, corticosteroid use, smokers.

4 If the patient is on an IV preparation, then all dental work should have been completed prior commencement of IV bisphosphonates.

5 If dental extractions are required and they are on IV then contact the patient's oncologist to discuss this further. Non-urgent procedures ideally need to be delayed for 3–6 months following interruption of bisphosphonate treatment (invasive procedures should be completed before initiation of high dose bisphosphonate). Patients on oral bisphosphonates have much lower

risk of BRONJ than those on IV but you may discuss with the prescribing physician the option of stopping bisphosphonates for 3 months, especially in those who have been on treatment for more than 3 years and/or have additional risk factors (for more information see the American Association of Oral & Maxillofacial Surgeons website, 'Bisphosphonates' Position Paper 2006 & Evidence-based Dentistry 2008).

6 Explain that you will carried out the extraction as carefully (atraumatic) as possible to keep the risk low.

7 Explain you may prescribing post-operative antibiotics.

8 They will need to be meticulous about their oral hygiene.

9 Inform the patient they will need follow-up until the socket has completely healed.

B Clotting defect

1 Explain to the patient that as they are on warfarin, which 'thins' their blood, they will bleed more after tooth extraction. However, it is often not necessary to stop the warfarin, so they should continue to take their usual warfarin dose. Therapeutic INR for atrial fibrillation is in the range of 2–2.5 and so long as their INR is less than 4, simple extractions can be carried out.
   - Ascertain what the range of their INR usually is and assess how much it fluctuates.
   - This can be done by checking their 'yellow' anticoagulant book.

2 Explain that the patient will need to have their INR check if possible on the morning of the extraction or the day before extraction. It is now possible to obtain an instant INR reading and GP practices often can provide this.

3 Is the patient taking any other medication which may also make them more prone to bleeding, eg anti-platelet agents (aspirin/clopidogrel).

4 Tell them that additional local measures will be taken:
   - Suturing of socket
   - Packing with an haemostatic agent, eg oxidised

cellulose, fibrin foam)
- Topical tranexamic acid (mouthwash) may be given in some cases.

5   Explain that if their INR is greater than 4 then it will be necessary to discuss this with their physician/ haematologist.

Comment

INR is the ratio of the patient's prothrombin time relative to the control prothrombin time. Normal INR is 1. Pain should be controlled with paracetamol/codeine analgesia. It is best to avoid NSAIDs. The use of antibiotics needs to considered carefully as some interfere with anticoagulation control.

C   Diabetes mellitus

1   Explain to the patient that treatment under local anaesthesia does not require adjustment to their diabetic treatment regimen but if they require sedation or a general anaesthetic, which involves being nil by mouth, they will need to make changes to their normal diabetic medication. These cases are best treated in hospital.

2   Explain that you do need some more information regarding their diabetes, such as:
- How well controlled is their diabetes? If it is tightly (or well) controlled there is a concern they may become hypoglycaemic during the extraction procedure.
- Are they diet-controlled, or are they taking oral hypoglycaemics or insulin?
- Do they have any associated medical problems, eg ischaemic heart disease, renal failure?

3   Explain about other concerns and additional measures for diabetes mellitus:
- Encourage the patient to eat their meals and medication at normal times.
- It is important to minimise the possibility of hypoglycaemia during the procedure, so you need to schedule the appointment to avoid interruption of normal mealtimes – morning is often better or just after lunchtime.

- It may be necessary for the patient to adjust their insulin dose, depending on their ability to eat following the extraction.
- It is important to provide instructions for good mouth care post-extraction to reduce risk of infections.
- Consider post-operative antibiotics as problems can arise with wound healing and secondary infection.
- Explain that people with diabetes do not tolerate infections well and their insulin requirements increase in response to infection. Should they develop an infection their blood glucose levels will be higher than usual and they need to seek medical attention.

Comment

Patients with diabetes (especially poorly controlled) are more prone to periodontal disease. They also have phagocytic dysfunction, though it is uncertain whether this leads to increase susceptibility to infections.

CHAPTER 10

DRUGS AND THERAPEUTICS

Chapter 10: Questions

OSCE Station 10.1
5 minute station

You are a dentist in practice and are about to administer intravenous sedation to a patient. You need to place an intravenous cannula. Using the mannequin arm, insert the cannula and explain your actions as you proceed.

Props:

- Mannequin arm
- Tourniquet
- Sterile wipe
- Adhesive dressing
- Cannula
- Saline flush
- Gloves
- Sharps bin

OSCE Station 10.2
5 minute station

Please prepare and give this antibiotic to the patient by intramuscular injection.

Props:

- Ampoule of benzylpenicillin powder
- Liquid for mixing
- Selection of needles
- Syringes
- Sterile wipe
- Cotton-wool swab
- Sharps bin

OSCE Station 10.3
5 minute station

You are an SHO in an oral and maxillofacial surgery unit. You have admitted an insulin-dependent diabetic patient to the ward, who is undergoing a bimaxillary osteotomy the next day. You need to place the patient on a sliding scale. Please explain how you would proceed.

OSCE Station 10.4
5 minute station

You are an SHO in an oral and maxillofacial surgery unit. You have seen a patient with atypical facial pain who is to be treated with gabapentin. Please write a prescription for the patient and explain to the patient how they should take this medication.

OSCE Station 10.5
5 minute station

Mr Smith is taking the following medications:

- Nifedipine
- Amitriptyline
- Amoxicillin
- Penicillamine
- Phenytoin

What are the possible oral side-effects of these preparations?

OSCE Station 10.6
5 minute station

You need to stock your emergency drug box/kit in your dental practice. Name six drugs you would order, in what doses/strengths you would order them and how you would administer them. Name one emergency when you would use each of the drugs that you have named.

OSCE Station 10.7
5 minute station

A   A petite, fit and healthy 18-year-old girl attends your surgery for extraction of her wisdom teeth. She weighs 47kg. What is the maximum dose of lidocaine with adrenaline (epinephrine) she may be given?

B   A frail 76-year-old woman requires multiple extractions but reports previous adverse reaction to lidocaine. What is the maximum dose of prilocaine she may be given.

C   What are the signs and symptoms of local anaesthetic overdose?

Chapter 10: Answers

OSCE Station 10.1

1 Introduce yourself politely to the patient.

2 Check the patient's identity.

3 Explain the procedure in a clear and succinct manner and gain their consent.

4 Check that the correct equipment is available before starting the procedure.

5 Put on the gloves.

6 Place the tourniquet on the arm.

7 Select an appropriate vein.

8 Clean the skin with an alcohol wipe.

9 Check the cannula.

10 Warn the patient of a sharp scratch.

11 Insert the needle at approximately 35–45°.

12 Look for flash-back into the cannula chamber.

13 Release the tourniquet.

14 Insert the cannula while withdrawing the introducer.

15 Put on the cap on the end of the cannula (to stop bleeding as the introducer is removed).

16 Secure the cannula with a dressing.

17 Flush the cannula with saline.

18 Dispose of sharps appropriately.

The entire procedure should be done in as fluent and as clean a manner as possible.

OSCE Station 10.2

1 Introduce yourself politely to the patient.

2 Check the patient's identity.

3 Explain the procedure in a clear and succinct manner.

4 Check the patient's medical history with respect to allergies and previous penicillin usage.

5 Check that the correct equipment is available before starting the procedure.

6 Obtain consent to proceed.

7 Put on the gloves.

8 Check the drug – quantity and use-by date, and whether it is appropriate for intramuscular usage.

9 Check the drawing-up liquid and its use-by date.

10 Clean the top of the ampoule with an alcohol wipe.

11 Inject the liquid into the ampoule.

12 Shake to allow the powder to dissolve; draw up into the syringe by inverting the ampoule.

13 Change to the injection needle.

14 Select the site for injection – deltoid or gluteal muscles can be used.

15 Clean the area with an alcohol wipe.

16 Pinch up the muscle and inject with a stabbing motion.

17 Aspirate to check that the needle is not in a blood vessel.

18 Inject the liquid.

19 Withdraw the needle and apply pressure to the wound.

20 Apply a plaster if needed.

21 Dispose of sharps appropriately.

The entire procedure should be done in a fluent manner.

Deltoid site

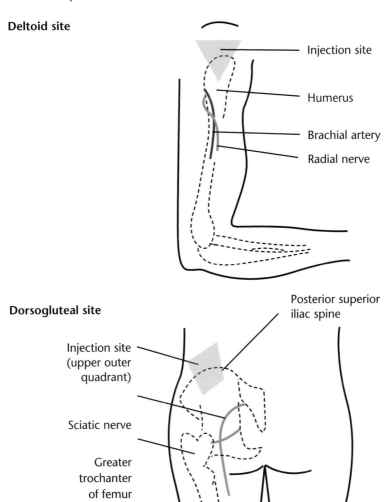

OSCE Station 10.3

1   Inform the anaesthetist and diabetic team of the admission.

2   Take the medical history to determine the patient's usual insulin regimen (type, quantity and timing of their regular insulin).

3   Get blood tests done: full blood count, urea and electrolytes, random glucose. If the results are acceptable, then the patient can take their normal insulin and carbohydrate intake up to the evening before the operation (including evening meal).

4   Explain that they need to omit their long-acting insulin on the day before the operation.

5   The patient needs to be fasted prior to a general anaesthetic so once this is commenced start a dextrose and insulin sliding scale. No single sliding scale will apply to all patients. A rough guideline is to divide the patient's total daily insulin requirement by 24, which gives the amount per hour (eg if the usual insulin requirement = 60 IU/day, infuse 60/24 = 2.5 IU/hour).

Blood glucose (BM) mmol/L	Units of insulin (Actrapid®)/hour	Additional instructions*
< 4.0	0.5	Inform SHO, stop infusion and give glucose/dextrose
4.1–8.0	1.0	↑ BM frequency
8.1–12.0	2.0	
12.1–16.0	3.5	
16.1–20.0	4.5	↑ BM frequency
> 20	6.0	Inform SHO

Table 10.3
*Additional instuctions are written on the drug chart for the nursing staff administering the drug.

6   Establish intravenous access to allow administration of the infusion.

7   Check the patient's blood glucose (BM; fingerprick test) prior
     to starting the infusion.

8   Continue the insulin/dextrose infusion until the patient is eating
     and drinking adequately.

Comment

Diabetic patients are more likely to have heart disease and renal
impairment and reduced resistance to infection. All diabetic
patients will require pre-operative investigations, including urea
and electrolytes, electrocardiography (ECG) and prophylactic antibiotics. Treat non-insulin-dependent diabetic patients in the same
way as insulin-dependent diabetic patients for anything other
than a short procedure. Patients treated under local anaesthesia
or local anaesthesia and sedation should maintain their carbohydrate intake and any oral hypoglycaemic drugs as usual and treatment should be planned to fit in with their regular mealtimes.
Have carbohydrate/sugars at hand if necessary.

Place non-insulin-dependent diabetic patients first on a list. The
patient should have their usual oral hypoglycaemic agents the
day before the operation. Omit oral hypoglycaemic agents and
breakfast on the day of operation. Check the BM first thing in the
morning and every 2 hours after that. Consider stopping long-
acting oral hypoglycaemic agents the day before operation.

OSCE Station 10.4

Mr Atypical Facial Pain

21 High Street, Thamestown, AB1 9RF

DOB: 3 September 1950

Gabapentin

Day 1 – 300 mg oral (OD)

Day 2 – 300 mg oral (BDS)

Day 3 – 300 mg oral (TDS)

Then increase according to response in steps of 300 mg (in three divided doses) to a maximum of 2.4 g per day

Please supply 100 tablets

Signature

Address

Date

Comment

- The explanation to the patient should include how to take the tablets, starting with 300 mg on day 1, two divided doses of 300 mg on day 2, three divided doses of 300 mg on day 3.
- The patient can then increase the dose by 300 mg a day to a maximum of eight tablets a day in three divided doses, if their pain is not controlled. The usual dose for pain control is between 900 mg and 1.2 g per day. The

patient may experience some side-effects when taking this drug, in particular, dizziness, somnolence, ataxia, nausea and vomiting.

OSCE Station 10.5

- Nifedipine – This is a calcium-channel blocker, which is mainly used as an antihypertensive agent. It can lead to gingival hyperplasia typically, with red and puffy papillae with a tendency to bleeding.
- Amitriptyline – This can cause dry mouth. Drugs with anticholinergic or sympathomimetic or diuretic activity can cause dry mouth. These include:
  - Atropine and hyoscine
  - Antidepressants, phenothiazines
  - Antihistamines
  - Anti-reflux agents, eg omeprazole
  - Opioids
  - Diuretics
- Amoxicillin – Broad-spectrum antibiotics can lead to *Candida* infections and antibiotic sore mouth, GI upset.
- Penicillamine – Anti-rheumatic drugs can lead to lichenoid reactions. (Other drugs that can cause lichenoid reactions include gold, antihypertensives [eg captopril, methyldopa, furosemide] and allopurinol.)
- Phenytoin – This is mainly used in the treatment of epilepsy. It can cause gingival enlargement/hyperplasia, which is typically firm and pale. Other drugs that cause gingival enlargement include nifedipine and ciclosporin.

OSCE Station 10.6

	Drug	Condition	Dose	Route
1	Glyceryl trinitrate	Acute angina	400 µg/dose	Spray sublingual
2	Salbutamol aerosol inhaler	Asthma	100 µg/ actuation	Inhalation
3	Aspirin, dispersible	Myocardial infarction	300 mg	Orally
4	Glucagon	Hypoglycaemic attack	1 mg	Intramuscularly
5	Midazolam	Status epilepticus	5 mg/mL or 10 mg/mL	Intranasal/ buccally
6	Adrenaline (epinephrine)	Anaphylactic reaction	1 mL of 1:1000, 1mg/mL	Intramuscularly
7	Glucose solution/ gel/tablets/ powder	Hypoglycaemic attack		Oral
8	Oxygen	Anaphylactic reaction, asthmatic attack, angina, myocardial infarction, cardiac arrest, epilepsy	10 L/min	Inhalation

Table 10.6

Comment

For more information regarding management of medical emergencies within the dental surgery please see the Resuscitation Council (UK) website (www.resus.org.uk).

OSCE Station 10.7

A The maximum safe dose of lidocaine with adrenaline
(epinephrine) is 7 mg/kg. The maximum dose is
7 x 47= 329 mg. Lidocaine in dental local anaesthetic comes
as lidocaine 2% with adrenaline (epinephrine) 1:80 000
usually in 2.2 mL cartridges. A 2% solution of any anaesthetic
solution translates to 20 mg/mL. So the maximum dose is
329/20 = 16.45 mL, ie seven (2.2 mL) cartridges of lidocaine
2% with adrenaline (epinephrine) 1:80 000. Also check in the
British National Formulary.

Local anaesthetic	Maximum safe dose	Average 70 kg/ maximum cartridges
Lidocaine with adrenaline (epinephrine)	7 mg/kg (500 mg in 70 kg)	11 cartridges of 2.2 mL
Lidocaine	4.5 mg/kg (300 mg in 70 kg)	
Prilocaine (3%) with felypressin	8 mg/kg	8 cartridges of 2.2 mL
Prilocaine	6 mg/kg	4 cartridges of 2.2 mL
Bupivacaine with adrenaline (epinephrine)	2 mg/kg	
Bupivacaine	2 mg/kg	

Table 10.7

B The maximum dose of prilocaine is stated above. As a
dental local anaesthetic, the formulation is prilocaine 4%
plain or prilocaine 3% with felypressin 0.3 IU or prilocaine
3% with adrenaline (epinephrine), 1:300 000. One needs to
take into consideration the weight of the patient, but reduce
the dose suitably as patient is elderly and frail. Aim to use the
minimum dose possible. In 4% prilocaine solution there is
40 mg/mL.

Comment

Cartridges come as 2.2 mL and 1.8 mL for lidocaine but as 1.8 mL for prilocaine. Remember, maximum quoted doses are for fit and healthy patients and so will need to be reduced in the elderly.

C   Signs and symptoms of local anaesthetic overdose:

Local anaesthetic agents are relatively free from side-effects if they are administered in an appropriate dosage and in the correct anatomical location. Systemic toxic effects due to local anaesthetics involve primarily the central nervous system and the cardiovascular system.

CNS signs and symptoms of local anaesthetic toxicity are:

- Early/mild toxicity: light-headedness, dizziness, circum-oral paraesthesia, visual and/or auditory disturbances such as difficulty focusing and tinnitus. Other subjective CNS symptoms include disorientation and drowsiness. Objective signs of CNS toxicity include shivering, muscular twitching and tremors initially involving muscles of the face and distal parts of the extremities.
- Severe toxicity: generalised convulsions of a tonic–clonic nature occur, may progress to generalised CNS depression and coma. Respiratory depression may result in respiratory arrest.

CVS signs and symptoms of local anaesthetic toxicity are:

- Early or mild toxicity: tachycardia and rise in blood pressure, if there is adrenaline (epinephrine) in the local anaesthetic. If no adrenaline (epinephrine) is added then bradycardia with hypotension will occur.
- Severe toxicity: collapse is due to the depressant effect of the local anaesthetic acting directly on the myocardium.

CHAPTER 11

LAW AND ETHICS

Chapter 11: Questions

OSCE Station 11.1
5 minute station

You are an SHO in an oral and maxillofacial surgery unit. You have to obtain consent from a 23-year-old man with learning difficulties for an examination under anaesthetic and extractions as necessary. He lives in a residential home and has attended with his carer.

A How will you obtain consent for this procedure?

B What does the law say about who may give consent for procedures?

C What types of consent are there?

OSCE Station 11.2
5 minute station

You are a senior partner in a dental practice. One of the practice dental nurses has come to talk to you. She is upset as she overheard a patient treated at the practice complaining in the waiting room that she thought her practitioner had been negligent.

A Please explain what negligence is, and what must be proved for a case to ensue with respect to dental care.

B Also explain what the difference is between contributory negligence and vicarious liability.

OSCE Station 11.3
5 minute station

You are a dentist in a new general dental practice. Please explain how your NHS complaints system should be set up.

OSCE Station 11.4
5 minute station

You are a dentist in practice who wishes to employ a dental hygienist. What documents would you wish to see to enable them to work in your practice.

OSCE Station 11.5
5 minute station

An 11-year-old girl, Chloe, attends the dental surgery with her aunt. She is on holiday staying with her aunt and cousins and they have been trampolining earlier in the day. Unfortunately Chloe fell off the trampoline and has fractured her upper left central incisor. You have requested a telephone number to contact Chloe's mother but her aunt wants to know why you need to do this as she is here with Chloe. Please explain to Chloe's aunt what are the issues surrounding consent for examination and treatment of Chloe?

OSCE Station 11.6
5 minute station

A   What is audit?

B   Why is it done?

C   Please fill in the audit cycle.

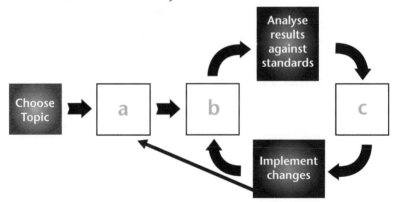

Chapter 11: Answers

OSCE Station 11.1

A No one can give consent on behalf of an adult person, even if the adult is incompetent. (Competence is defined as the ability to perform a task, which in this case is to make a decision.) You will therefore need to obtain consent from the patient in question. The severity of his learning difficulties will determine how and what the patient understands. If the patient does have some degree of understanding, you will need to explain the procedure in a way that he can understand.

B If the patient cannot understand, it is obvious that treatment may need to be given which is in the best interest of the patient, and his inability to consent to the treatment should not prevent the treatment from being given. Only such treatment that is in the best interest of the patient should be carried out. In these situations information should be sought from the relatives and carers of the patient, and it is useful to have the agreement of those close to the patient to carry out treatment although this is not consent.

C Consent may be 'express', in which case the patient explicitly agrees to treatment, and it may be oral or written. The General Dental Council requires that written consent is gained for the administration of sedation or general anaesthesia, but in many hospitals consent forms are used for all surgical procedures. In certain situations it may be advisable for two doctors/dentists to sign a consent form for treatment in the patient's best interest. 'Implied' consent is when you assume from a patient's conduct that they have consented – sitting in a dental chair, for example is taken to mean that the patient consents to an examination.

OSCE Station 11.2

A Negligence is failure to exercise reasonable care in one's professional capacity. This obviously depends on what reasonable care means, but so long as a dentist can show that they acted in line with what most of his or her colleagues would have done it is unlikely that they would be held negligent. For negligence to be proved it must be shown that the dentist had a duty of care to the patient, that there was a breach of that duty and that this resulted in damage to the patient.

B 'Contributory negligence' is when the patient has contributed to the damage, such as when they have not followed the dentist's instructions. 'Vicarious liability' is when an employer is held responsible for the actions of anyone in their employ (eg a dental nurse) although that employee will also be held responsible for their own actions.

OSCE Station 11.3

Points to cover:

- Each practice must have a complaints procedure, with one person being in charge of its administration.
- The practice complaints procedure must be available to the patients.
- All records relating to a complaint must be kept, but should not be stored in the patient's notes.
- Patients have 6 months from the time of the incident to complain or 6 months from the time they noticed a problem, provided this is less than 12 months after the incident.
- On receiving a complaint, a written acknowledgement must be made within 2 working days.
- Following investigation of the complaint, a written response should be sent to the patient within 10 working days of the original complaint.
- If the patient is not satisfied with the outcome they can ask the local primary care trust to look into the matter.

Possible outcomes following this are:

- The complaint is referred back to the practice.
- Conciliation.
- Independent review panel of a convener and two independent members.
- Healthcare commission.
- Advising the patient to contact the Health Services Ombudsman.
- No further action.

OSCE Station 11.4

- A dentist may legally designate almost all non-surgical management of periodontal disease to a dental hygienist or a dual-qualified dental therapist, provided they are registered.
- As an employer you would want to have seen the following documents:
  - General Dental Council (GDC) annual practising certificate
  - Current membership of a dental defence organisation to allow for indemnity against claims for professional negligence
  - Any post-qualification certificates allowing the hygienist to carry out radiography, administer local anaesthetic, etc
  - Evidence of updating of basic life support skills with in the last 12 months
  - Evidence of immunisation against hepatitis B
  - Evidence of continuing professional development
  - Evidence from the criminal records bureau of a clean record

Comment

The principal dentist in a practice has the responsibility to comply with employment legislation and GDC guidelines. Up-to-date records of staff must be kept, along with current practising certificates. Annual verification of professional indemnity insurance and basic life support skills must be kept. It is also necessary to ensure that all professionals complementary to dentistry (PCDs) work within the code of professional conduct and competencies according to the GDC curricula.

CHAPTER 11
Answers

OSCE Station 11.5

1   Explain that Chloe is a minor and the currently accepted age of consent in the UK is 16, provided the individual has the capacity (ie intelligence maturity and understanding). If they do not, then the age of consent is 18. However, there is the issue of 'Gillick competence' – this is where a minor can consent for themselves, provided they have capacity. Also, the proposed treatment must be in the minor's best interests and every reasonable effort must have been made to involve the parents or legal guardian of the minor. Chloe is still very young to consent for complex dental treatment by herself (although she probably would be able to consent to an examination), so every effort should be made to contact whoever has parental responsibility for Chloe. If contact cannot be made it would and it is an absolute emergency then treatment:
- Must not be denied to Chloe
- Must be in her best interests

2   It may also be advantageous to involve another colleague in the practice to confirm that treatment was absolutely necessary and was in Chloe's best interests.

3   The treatment should be explained and agreed by her aunt.

4   If possible only reversible treatment rather than anything such as an extraction should be carried out and further treatment only given when parental consent has been gained.

5   Ask Chloe's aunt if she has any questions.

302 OSCES FOR DENTISTRY

OSCE Station 11.6

A   Audit is a systematic examination of current practice to assess how well an institution or practitioner is performing against set standards. It is a method for systematically reflecting on, reviewing and improving practice. Areas of deficiency can be identified and remedied.

B   The main purpose of audit is to increase the quality of service/care provided to users (patients). It identifies and promotes good practice, and can lead to improvement in service delivery and outcome for users. An audit helps provide information about the effectiveness of the service and provides an opportunity for training and education. It also helps ensure efficiency by ensuring better use of resources.

C   Audit cycle

(a)   Set standard
(b)   Collect data
(c)   Identify changes to be made

MOCK OSCES

Chapter 12: Questions

OSCE Station 12.1
5 minute station

Please look at these lesions and indicate which type of biopsy is indicated for each and what you think the lesions are.

a

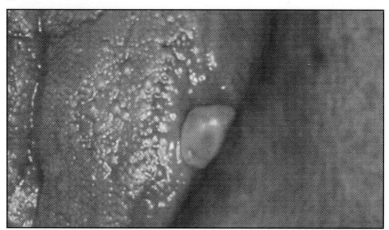

b

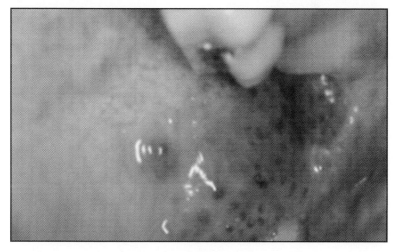

c

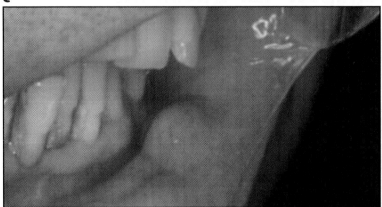

d

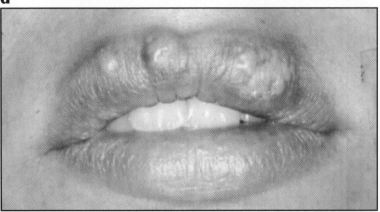

e

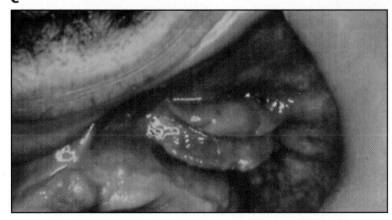

f

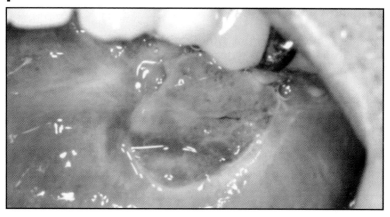

OSCE Station 12.2
5 minute station

A   Describe the clinical signs seen in this photograph.

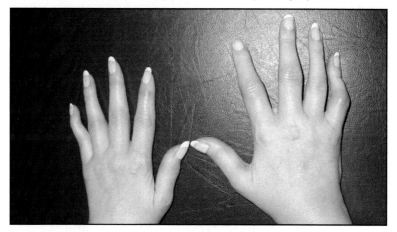

B   What medical condition does the patient have?

C   How may this condition influence dental treatment and health?

OSCE Station 12.3
10 minute station

You are about to carry out a surgical procedure for this patient. Please don the protective gear, wash your hands and put on the sterile gloves ready to carry out the surgical procedure.

Props:

- Safety glasses
- Mask
- Gown
- Sterile gloves
- Hand-washing facilities

OSCE Station 12.4
5 minute station

You are a dentist in practice who has just had a needlestick injury in your finger.

How should you proceed and what steps should be covered?

OSCE Station 12.5
5 minute station

A 23-year-old woman has attended your practice with pericoronitis.

A Please write a prescription for metronidazole along with ibuprofen for pain relief for this patient.

B What information do you need about the patient in order to write the prescription and what information would you provide to the patient?

Pharmacy stamp		Age	Name (including forename) and address	
		DOB		
Dispenser's endorsement	Number of days treatment NB Ensure dose is stated		NP	Pricing Office
Pack & Quantity				
Signature of Dentist			Date	
For dispenser No. of prescns on form	Dentist's name and address			

OSCE Station 12.6

5 minute station

Please take a history from this patient regarding their complaint of a swelling in the submandibular region.

OSCE Station 12.7
5 minute station

A patient attends your dental practice seeking advice on whether she can have her fractured upper central incisor restored. On examination, the tooth is fractured, with inadequate coronal tooth tissue to fabricate a crown on. The tooth has a good root canal filling in place with no evidence of periapical pathology.

Please discuss the treatment options with the patient.

OSCE Station 12.8
5 minute station

A patient presents with a 1-cm-diameter lump in their palate.

What is the differential diagnosis and what investigations would you carry out?

OSCE Station 12.9
5 minute station

Please fill in the missing items in this table of emergency drugs.

Condition	Drug	Dose	Route of administration
	Adrenaline (epinephrine)		Intramuscular
Anaphylaxis	Hydrocortisone		
Hypoglycaemia			Oral
Hypoglycaemia			IIntramuscular
Epileptic fit		5–10 mg	
Chest pain	GTN		
Acute asthma			Inhaler

Table 12.9a

OSCE Station 12.10
5 minute station

You are a dentist in general practice and have just fitted a partial denture for a patient who has not worn dentures before.

What instructions would you give them?

OSCE Station 12.11
5 minute station

A colleague has carried out some research using a new mouthwash to detect dysplasia in intra-oral white patches. The results are shown below:

Mouthwash result	Dysplastic white patch	Non-dysplastic white patch	Total
Positive result	20	11	31
Negative result	4	125	129
Total	24	136	160

Table 12.11

However, they have been asked to calculate some simple statistics on the results and they do not know how to do this. Please help them work out these particular values for them:

1 How many true positives are there?

2 How many false negatives are there?

3 What do you understand by the terms sensitivity and specificity?

4 What is the sensitivity of this test?

5 What is the specificity of this test?

6 What is the positive predictive value of this test?

7 What is the negative predictive value of this test?

OSCE Station 12.12
5 minute station

You have taken a lower alginate impression to make a soft bite-raising appliance. Please disinfect the impression and fill in the laboratory card to send the impression to the laboratory.

Props:

- Alginate impression in a lower tray
- Sink and running water
- Bath for disinfection with appropriate solution
- Laboratory card
- Plastic bag
- Tissue/gauze

Chapter 12: Answers

OSCE Station 12.1

(a) Excisional biopsy – This is a fibroepithelial polyp.

(b) No biopsy – This is a haemangioma.

(c) Excisional biopsy – This is a mucocoele.

(d) No biopsy – This is herpes labialis.

(e) Excisional biopsy – This is a denture granuloma.

(f) Incisional biopsy – This is a tongue ulcer which could be a squamous-cell carcinoma.

OSCE Station 12.2

A The clinical signs seen in the photograph are:

- Fingers with swanneck deformity (hyperextended proximal interphalangeal [PIP] joints and flexed distal interphalangeal [DIP] joints).
- Boutonnière's deformity (flexed PIP joints, extended metacarpophalangeal [MCP] joints and hyperextended DIP joints).
- Other features associated with rheumatoid arthritis but not seen on this picture are thumbs with 'Z' deformities and subluxation of the MCP joints and wrists with ulnar deviation.

B Rheumatoid arthritis.

C
- The patient may be on non-steroidal anti-inflammatory drugs (NSAIDs), so you do not want to prescribe further NSAIDs for dental pain.

- The patient may be on steroids. Consider the need for prophylaxis in those with actual or potential adrenocortical suppression. Dose for prophylaxis is 100 mg hydrocortisone (as sodium succinate) intramuscularly, 30 minutes pre-operatively.
- The patient may have rheumatoid arthritis in other joints, eg temporomandibular joints.
- The patient may have other problems, eg the rheumatoid arthritis may be part of a connective tissue disorder in Sjögren's syndrome.
- The patient may have difficulty with toothbrushing due to decreased manual dexterity.
- If the patient is to have a general anaesthetic there is a risk of atlanto-axial joint subluxiation when extending the neck.

CHAPTER 12
Answers

OSCE Station 12.3

1   Open the pack with the gown inside, but do not touch anything inside. Then open the sterile glove packet and drop the gloves onto the gown, all prior to washing.

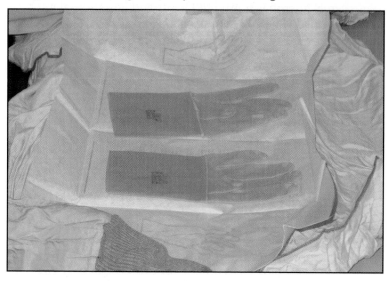

2   Put on the mask and safety glasses before you start to wash and don the sterile clothing.

3   Remove jewellery and watches from the fingers and wrists.

4   Set the water flow and temperature to the right level.

5   Wash your hands and forearms thoroughly, going from fingertips to elbows with a surgical hand-scrub.

6   Brush your nails (and not skin) with the nailbrush, while leaving wet soap on your hands and forearms to work. After about a minute of nail-scrubbing, discard the brush and wash your hands thoroughly, going from fingers to elbows.

7   Do not turn the taps off with your clean hands – use your elbows.

8 Dry your hands on the sterile towel in the gown packet, going from fingers to elbows.

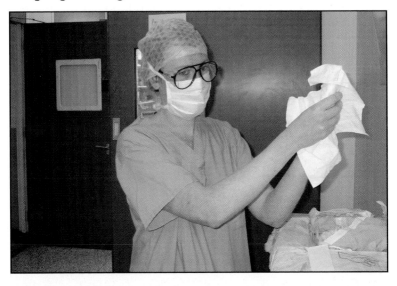

9 Place gown on without touching the sterile front surface.

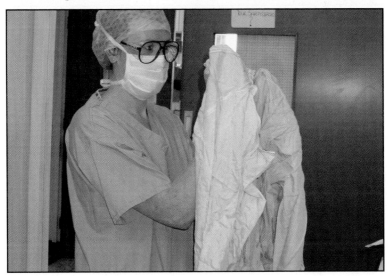

10 Allow the assistant to tie the back of the gown up. Do not put your hands behind your back to tie the gown up.

11 Put on the gloves without touching the fingers of the gloves with your fingers.

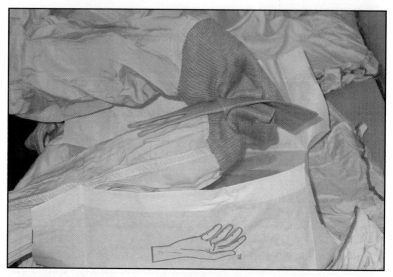

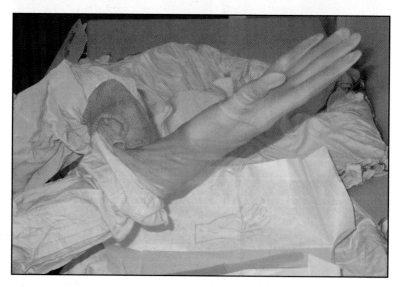

OSCE Station 12.4

Points to cover:

- First aid.
- Encourage the wound to bleed.
- Wash the area with water and soap, but do not scrub the wound.
- Cover it with a waterproof dressing.
- If the treatment can be stopped at this point, then stop the treatment.
- If possible, another member of staff should assess the viral carrier status of the source patient, and hence the likely risk of transmission of an infectious disease.
- Local arrangements should be in place at the practice to enable follow-up action to be carried out.
- The incident should be recorded in the practice accident book. Details recorded should include:
    - Who was injured?
    - How has the accident occurred?
    - What action was taken?
    - Who was informed and when?
    - Who was the source patient ?
- Each primary care trust will have at least one designated specialist (often the consultant medical microbiologist) who can be contacted for advice on post-exposure prophylaxis. Details of how to contact them should be clearly displayed in the dental practice.
- If there is a worry that the source patient may be high-risk for an infectious disease, then urgent advice should be sought according to the local rules (see above). This may involve going to the nearest accident and emergency department, where you must have the following checked:
    - Tetanus status – If inadequate, a tetanus booster will be needed.
    - Hepatitis B status – If previously immunised, anti body titres should be checked. If low, a booster vaccine is needed; if very low, then immunoglobulins will be needed and a vaccine course should be started. If not previously immunised (this should not be the case for healthcare workers in the UK), hepatitis B immunoglobulins should be given and an active immunisation course started (first vaccine

in accident and emergency and arrangements made for subsequent doses).
- If the source patient is known to be human immunodeficiency virus (HIV) positive, or hepatitis C positive, immediate specialist advice must be sought, and antiretroviral drugs taken prophylactically as soon as possible.
- Baseline bloods may be required from the source patient for storage and possible future testing. This will have to be done by another healthcare professional to avoid conflict of interest, and only after proper consent has been obtained from the patient.
- Counselling and follow-up should be arranged as necessary.

Comment

Risk of acquiring hepatitis B following a needlestick injury from a carrier has been estimated at 2–40%; the risk of hepatitis C is believed to be 3–10%. The risk of acquiring HIV after a needlestick injury from an HIV-positive source is 0.2–0.5% but may be higher if significant volumes have been injected.

OSCE Station 12.5

A Points to cover are as follows:

1 Check that patient is not allergic to either medicine.

2 Check whether the patient is taking any other medication that may interfere with what you are about to prescribe. Note that the patient may be on the oral contraceptive pill, and should be advised to take other precautions as the antibiotics may upset the gastrointestinal absorption of the pill.

3 Check that the patient is not pregnant.

4 Check that the patient is not asthmatic or if she has any gastrointestinal bleeding which would contraindicate ibuprofen.

5 Advise the patient not to drink alcohol with the metronidazole.

B The prescription:

- Must be written legibly in ink
- Must be dated
- Must have the patient's full name and address
- Should have the age of the patient and give her date of birth. (It is only a legal requirement in the case of pre-scription-only medicines to state the age of children under 12 years.)
- Must be signed in ink by the prescriber
- Should have the names of the drugs written out in full
- Should have the quantity to be supplied stated, by indi-cating the number of days the treatment is required for.

Pharmacy stamp		Age 23 DOB 2.3.1982	Name (including forename) and address Poppy Patient Flat 1, 20 High Street, Thamestown, AZ1 2BX	
Dispenser's endorsement	Number of days treatment NB Ensure dose is stated	5 days	NP	Pricing Office
Pack & Quantity	Metronidazole, 400 mg oral, three times daily for 5 days. Total of 15 tablets. Avoid alcohol. Ibuprofen 400 mg oral, three times daily for 5 days. Total 15 tablets. Take with food.			
Signature of Dentist *A N Other*			Date 2.5.2005	
For dispenser No. of prescns on form	Dentist's name and address Dr A.N. Other, Smiles Dental Practice, 89, Main Street, Thamestown, AZ7 2GC			

OSCE Station 12.6

1   Introduce yourself politely to the patient.

2   Presenting complaint – You need to determine the patient's chief complaint, so start by asking them what the problem is or why they came to see you today. Record their complaint in their own words.

3   History of presenting complaint – You then want to know all about the character and history of the swelling, so ask the patient to tell you about their swelling. Stick to open questions if possible. You will need to ask them about the following:

- Site
- Onset
- Does the swelling come and go?
- If so, how often and how long does it take to come and go?
- Any associated factors with the onset, eg association with eating?
- Is it enlarging/shrinking/staying the same as time goes by?
- Pain (it is easy to remember all the necessary questions by using the acronym 'PQRST–EAR'):

    Position
    Quality
    Radiation
    Site
    Timing
    Exacerbating factors
    Associated factors
    Relieving factors

- Exacerbating and relieving factors
- Previous treatment
- Associated features – redness, inflammation, bad taste in the mouth
- Difficulty swallowing or pain on swallowing
- Systemic upset, eg fever

OSCE Station 12.7

1   Introduce yourself politely to the patient.

2   Ask the patient what her main concerns are and what she wants from the restoration.

3   Check the patient's smile line.

4   The options to discuss include:

- Post core and crown
- Removal of the root and restore with a partial denture
- Removal of the root and restore with a bridge
- Removal of the root and dental implant

	Advantages	Disadvantages
Post core and crown	Fixed restoration If it fails, still have other options available	Risk of root fracture May require gingival recontouring
Removal of root and partial denture	Quick procedure Easy to make and cheap	Removable prosthesis Loss of the root can lead to bone loss so will require relining following alveolar remodelling
Removal of root and adhesive bridge Fixed restoration	No gingival coverage Cantilever design is possible	Removal of tooth substance of adjacent teeth Wings may interfere with deep overbite Bond may fail Difficult to mask the space beneath the pontic
Removal of root and implant	Fixed restoration Good aesthetics Hopefully permanent	Expensive Time-consuming Needs temporary replacement during integration

Table 12.7

OSCE Station 12.8

The easiest way to reach a differential diagnosis for any lesion is to use a 'surgical sieve'. Many different types are available. For example, you can use the acronym 'vitamin C' or the different layers of tissue at that site.

	Type of lesion	Example
V	Vascular	Haemangioma
I	Inflammatory/infective	Dental abscess, odontogenic cysts
T	Traumatic	Denture granuloma
A	Autoimmune	Bullous disorder
M	Metabolic	
I	Iatrogenic/idiopathic	Haematoma
N	Neoplastic (benign/malignant)	Squamous-cell carcinoma, salivary gland tumours, odontogenic tumours, Wegener's granulomatosis
C	Congenital/ developmental	Unerupted tooth, tori, hamartomas, nasopalatine cyst

Table 12.8a

Tissue layer	Example lesions
Epithelium	Squamous-cell carcinoma, odontogenic cysts, tumours
Connective tissue	Denture granuloma, fibroepithelial polyp, odontogenic tumours, salivary gland tumours
Periosteum	
Bone	Torus, osteogenic tumours
Nasal cavity – midline	
Maxillary sinus – lateral	Squamous-cell carcinoma from epithelial lining of sinus
Teeth/supporting structures	Unerupted tooth, dental abscess, eruption cyst

Table 12.8b

Investigations

You would carry out a thorough history and examination prior to carrying out any investigations, which:

- Vitality testing of associated teeth
- Percussion testing of associated teeth
- Radiographs, intra-oral/extra-oral
- Biopsy:
  - Punch biopsy
  - Incisional biopsy
  - Excisional biopsy
- Blood tests (eg for neoplastic lesions and autoimmune lesions)
- Further imaging – computed tomography (CT), magnetic resonance imaging (MRI)

OSCE Station 12.9

Condition	Drug	Dose	Route of administration
Anaphylaxis	Adrenaline (epinephrine) 0.5 ml of	1:1000 (500 micrograms)	Intramuscular
Anaphylaxis	Hydrocortisone	100–500 mg	Intramuscular/slow intravenous
Hypoglycaemia	Glucose drink	1–2 teaspoonfuls	Oral
Hypoglycaemia	Glucagon	1 mg	Intramuscular
Epileptic fit	Diazepam	5–10 mg	Intravenous (intramuscular / PR)
Chest pain	GTN	2 sprays/1 tablet	Sublingual
Acute asthma	Salbutamol	2 puffs	Inhaler

Table 12.9b

OSCE Station 12.10

- The patient should be shown how to insert and remove the denture. This should be done in front of a mirror and continued until you are happy that the patient will be able to insert and remove the denture on their own.
- Other instructions should be given in writing as well as verbally as patients often do not take in all the information given to them.
- Dentures must be kept clean, ideally after each meal. Brushing of the dentures is better than just soaking and can be done with a soft brush and soap. It is not necessary to clean them with excessively hot water and this should be avoided – in fact cold water is adequate. Proprietary cleaners can be used but are not necessary.
- Dentures should not be worn at night. This is important as the oral mucosa or 'skin of the mouth' needs time to recover. Wearing of the dentures at night might cause the patient to develop an infection of the soft tissue of the mouth. When the dentures are left out they should be kept moist as drying may cause warping.
- Eating will be strange to start off with. Therefore, cut food into small pieces and chew slowly for the initial period. They should only attempt chewy or sticky foods after they have mastered controlling the dentures.
- It is possible that the dentures may rub – rather like a new pair of shoes. This is common and can usually be easily remedied by some careful grinding or adjustment. However, the patient should not try to adjust them themselves.
- Inform the patient that you plan to review the denture in 7–10 days. If they are sore they should leave the denture out and if they are unable to wait until the review appointment they should make an earlier one. Ideally, they should re-insert the denture, either the day before or the morning of the appointment, so that the sore area can be seen.
- Also advise them to keep the review appointment even if they feel there are no problems, so that you can examine them.
- Ask them if they have any questions.

OSCE Station 12.11

1   True positives = 20

2   False negatives = 4

3   Sensitivity is the proportion of true positives that are correctly identified and specificity is the proportion of true negatives that are correctly identified. So in this case, specificity is the proportion of individuals free of dysplasia according to the test who had a negative mouthwash result. Sensitivity is the proportion of individuals out of those with a diagnosis of dysplasia who had a positive mouthwash result.

4   Sensitivity = 20/24 = 83.3%.

5   Specificity = 125/136 = 91.9%.

6   The positive predictive value is the probability that an individual who has a positive test result has the disease, so in this case of the 31 individuals who had a positive result only 20 had dysplasia, so the positive predictive value is = 20/31 = 64.5%.

7   The negative predictive value is the probability that someone who has a negative test result does not have the disease. So in this case of the 129 individuals who had a negative result, 125 did not have dysplasia so the negative predictive value is 125/129 = 96.9%.

OSCE Station 12.12

1   Rinse the impression under running water to remove blood and saliva.

2   Set up the disinfection bath with appropriate solution – usually a hypochlorite solution or perborate solution proprietary brand. Check disinfection time with the solution used.

3   Place the impression into the disinfectant bath and note the time, most solutions need 10 minutes of soaking.

4   While soaking fill in the laboratory card:

  • Fill in patient's details – name, date of birth (and hospital number if appropriate), address if needed
  • Next appointment date so work can be ready for appointment
  • Your name and address of dental surgery
  • Laboratory instructions – 'please cast up impression and make a lower soft bite-raising appliance'
  • Most laboratory cards have a box to fill in to verify decontamination, so fill in as necessary.
    After a couple of minutes of soaking, the examiner will ask you to continue as though the impression had been soaking for 10 minutes.
    1   Rinse impression and shake off excess water.
    2   Wrap in damp tissue or gauze, and place in plastic bag labelled with patients details.
    3   Attach laboratory card to bag with impression.

INDEX

Locators are by chapter number/station number.

A

abducens nerve 1.3
abrasion 4.4
abscesses
    in diabetics 5.7
    treatment for 6.3
accessory nerve 1.3
aciclovir 6.3, 6.9
adrenaline 9.3, 10.7, 12.9
airway obstruction 9.6
airway tubes 9.7
allergic reactions 9.3, 12.9
amalgam restorations 4.8
American-style suckers 5.12
amitriptyline 10.5
amoxicillin 6.3, 10.5
amphotericin B 6.3
anaemia 6.2
anaesthesia
    general 5.6, 5.17, 9.8, 12.2
    local 5.3, 5.6, 5.16, 10.7
analgesia 5.4
anaphylaxis 9.3, 12.9
anatomy 8.6, 8.7, 8.8
    cephalometry 2.3, 2.4
antibiotics
    for LJP 3.6
    metronidazole 12.5
    side-effects 4.16, 10.5
    for various conditions 6.3
antiviral agents 6.3, 6.9
aphthous ulcers 6.2
apical root fracture 2.8
arthritis 10.5, 12.2
asthma 9.3, 12.9
attrition 4.4
atypical facial pain 1.1

audit 11.5
autoimmune disorders 6.5, 7.4
avulsion 2.7, 2.12, 2.13

B

basic life support 9.1
Basic Periodontal Examination (BPE) 3.7
biopsy procedures 12.1
    fibroepithelial polyps 6.11, 12.1
    immune-mediated disease 7.4
    for Sjögren's syndrome 6.5
    suspected malignancy 5.1, 12.1
bisphosphonates 9.9
bleaching of teeth 4.11, 4.16
bleeding
    following tooth extraction 5.4, 9.9
    of gums 3.8
blisters 7.4
    see also stomatitis; ulcers
blood
    taking samples 9.4
    see also bleeding
blood pressure 9.5
body mass index (BMI) 9.8
bone nibblers 5.12
bottle caries 2.11
Boutonnière's deformity 12.2
Bowdler Henry Rake retractors 5.12
bridges 3.5, 3.10, 4.19, 12.7
    conventional 3.5
    resin 3.5
    see also dentures
brushing teeth 3.2
bruxism 1.2, 4.4
bulimia 4.4

C

Campbell's lines 8.5
cancer
    diagnosis 1.4, 6.6
    malignant ulcers 5.1, 5.2, 12.1
    precancerous lesions 6.12
Candida albicans 4.3
candidosis, chronic hyperplastic 7.7
canine teeth
    impacted 2.5
    radiography 2.5, 8.1, 8.2
    unerupted 8.2
cannulation 10.1
caries 2.14
    nursing 2.11
    prevention
        dietary advice 2.1, 2.11
        fluoride 2.2
        sealants 2.14
    treatment
        rampant caries 2.11
        restoration materials 4.8
cementoblastoma 8.11
cement preparation
    glass ionomer 4.10
    zinc phosphate 4.1
cement preparations
    glass ionomer 4.10
    zinc sulphate 4.1
cephalometric measurements 2.4
cephalometric radiograph 2.3
cephalometry 2.3, 2.4
check-ups on new patients 1.6
cheilitis, angular 6.3
chlorhexidine 3.2
cold sores 6.3, 6.9, 12.1
communication skills
    concerning extractions 5.3, 5.4,
    5.5, 5.8, 5.17
    lifestyle advice 2.1, 6.1
    obtaining consent 5.3, 6.10
    oral hygiene advice 3.2
    patients 5.6, 5.9, 6.8, 6.9, 10.4, 12.10

    providing medical information to
    written (to health professionals)
    5.2, 7.1, 12.5, 12.12
    see also history-taking
complaints procedures 11.3
composite restorations 4.8
computed tomography (CT) 8.8
consent
    legal issues 11.1, 11.5
    polyp removal 6.10
    tooth extraction 5.3
cores *see* posts
Coupland's chisels 5.12
cranial nerves 1.3
crossbite 2.16
crowns
    dentine-bonded 4.16
    fitting 4.17
    fractured 2.9
    gold 4.18
    partial jacket 4.16
    pericoronitis 12.5
    restoration 4.11, 12.7
CT (computed tomography) scans 8.8
Cvek pulpotomy 2.9
cysts
    mucocoeles 7.5, 12.1
    in the neck 1.4
    odontogenic keratocyst 7.3

D

dams 4.14
decay *see* caries
deciduous teeth *see* primary teeth
deltoid muscle 10.2
dental check-up 1.6
    children 2.1
dental hygienists 11.4
dental panoramic tomography 8.7,
8.10
dentures 3.10
    advantages/disadvantages 3.10, 12.7

granuloma 12.1
instructions to patient 12.10
partial 3.5, 4.19
stomatitis 4.3, 6.3
study models 4.15
see also bridges
diabetes 9.9
abscesses 5.7
hypoglycaemia 12.9
pre-operative preparation 10.3
tooth replacement 3.10
diagnosis
lumps and swellings 1.4, 7.5, 12.8
other lesions 6.6, 6.7, 6.12, 7.3, 7.4, 7.6, 7.8, 8.10
on pathology request forms 7.1
toothache 3.3
diazepam 9.2, 12.9
diet
excessive wear on teeth 4.4
reduction of dental decay 2.1, 2.11
dietary advice 2.1
diplopia 1.5
discoloration of teeth 2.7, 4.11, 4.16
disinfection 12.12
dry mouth 6.4, 6.5, 10.5
dysplasia 6.12, 7.8, 12.11

periapical lesions 3.3
posts and cores 4.12
pulpotomy 2.9, 2.10
vitality testing 4.13
endotracheal tubes 9.7
enophthalmos 1.5
epilepsy
drugs for 10.5, 12.9
fits 9.2
equipment 10.3
identification of 3.7, 5.12, 9.7
used for suturing 5.10
see also specific items
eruption *see* unerupted teeth
erythromycin 6.3
ethyl chloride vitality test 4.13
exophthalmus 1.5
extraction
obtaining consent 5.3
post-operative instructions 5.4
pre-operative counselling 5.5, 5.8, 5.17, 10.7
supernumerary teeth 2.6
eye
lacrimal gland flow rate test 6.5
orbital floor fracture 8.8
swelling 1.5
testing 1.5

E

electric pulp testers 4.13
emergency kit 10.6
employment issues 11.4
enamel
hypoplasia 4.16
loss 4.4
enamel matrix derivatives 3.4
endodontics
fractured teeth 2.8, 2.9, 12.7
iatrogenic damage 4.5, 4.6, 4.7
isolation methods 4.14

F

facebows 4.2
facial nerve 1.3
facial pain 1.1, 10.4
facial weakness 1.3
fainting 9.1
ferric sulphate 2.10
fibroepithelial polyps
biopsy 6.11, 12.1
consent for removal 6.10
fingers, arthritis in 12.2
fissure sealants 2.14
fits 9.2, 12.9

flossing 3.2
fluconazole 6.3
fluoride 2.2
fluoride supplements 2.2
fluorosis 4.16
formocresol 2.10
fractures
    incisors 2.8, 2.9, 11.5, 12.7
    mandible 1.8, 8.4
    orbital floor 8.8
    zygoma 8.5
furcation involvement in periodontal
disease 3.4

G

gabapentin 10.4
gastric reflux 4.4
giant cells 7.6
gingival hyperplasia 10.5
gingivitis
    antibiotic use 6.3
    necrotising ulcerative 3.1
    in pregnancy 3.8
    ulcerative 3.1
    see also periodontal lesions
gingivostomatitis 6.3
    herpetic 6.3
    hyperplasia 10.5
    see also periodontal lesions
glass ionomer cement 4.10
glossopharyngeal nerve 1.3
glucose 12.9
gluteal muscle 10.2
glyceryl trinitrate 12.9
granuloma 12.1
grinding (bruxism) 1.2, 4.4
Guedal airways 9.7
gums
    bleeding 3.8
    see also gingivitis
gums gingivitis 3.1, 3.8, 6.3
gutta percha vitality test 4.13

H

haemangioma 12.1
haemosiderin 7.6
health and safety
    needlestick injuries 12.4
    radiation protection 8.9
healthy eating 2.1
heart valve, prosthetic 5.16
Heimlich manoeuvre 9.6
hepatitis 12.4
herpes labialis 6.3, 6.9, 12.1
histology
    giant-cell lesions 7.6
    lichen planus 7.2
    mucus extravasation cyst 7.5
    odontogenic keratocyst 7.3
    request forms 7.1
history-taking
    facial pain 1.1
    routine check-up 1.6
    submandibular swelling 12.6
    ulcers 5.1
HIV 12.4
Howarth's periosteal elevators 5.12
human resources issues 11.4
hydrocortisone 12.2, 12.9
hypersensitivity 9.3, 12.9
hypoglobus 1.5
hypoglossal nerve 1.3
hypoglycaemia 12.9

I

ibuprofen 12.5
immunofluorescence 7.4
impacted teeth 2.5
impaction 2.5
implants 3.5, 3.10, 12.7
    single-tooth 3.5

see also re-implantation
impressions 12.12
incisors
    apical root fracture 2.8
    avulsion 2.7, 2.12, 2.13
    crown fracture 2.9
    delayed eruption 2.6
    drifting 3.6
    fractured 2.8, 2.9, 12.7
    missing 2.6, 2.16, 3.5
    unerupted 2.6
infections
    C. albicans 4.3
    diagnosis 6.6
    referral 5.7
    see also antibiotics
injections, intramuscular 10.2
instruments see equipment
insulin 10.3
intramuscular injections 10.2
intravenous line placement 10.1
isolation methods 4.14

J

jaw *see* mandible

K

keratocyst 7.3

L

lacrimal gland flow rate 6.5
laryngeal mask airways 9.7
Laster's retractors 5.12
lateral pterygoid muscle 1.2
legal issues
    complaints procedures 11.3
    consent 11.1
    employment practices 11.4
    negligence 11.2
    radiation protection 8.9
lichenoid reactions 6.7, 10.5
lichen planus 6.7, 6.8, 7.2
lidocaine 10.7
life support techniques 9.1
lips
    angular cheilitis 6.3
    herpes labialis 6.3, 6.9, 12.1
    mucocoele 7.5, 12.1
    salivary gland biopsy 6.5
localised juvenile periodontitis (LJP) 3.6
lower root forceps 5.12
lumps 9.1
    diagnosis 7.5, 12.8
    examination 1.4
    eye 1.5
    history-taking 12.6
    neck 1.4

M

malocclusion 1.8
mandible
    cephalometric points 2.3
    clicking 5.15
    dislocation 5.11
    fracture 1.8, 8.4
    giant-cell lesions 7.6
    jaw opening exercises 5.13
    locking 5.15
    movement of 1.2, 4.9, 5.13
    pain on movement 5.9
    radiolucent lesions 8.10
    trauma 1.7
    see also temporomandibular joints
masticatory system examination 1.2
medicolegal issues *see* legal issues
metronidazole 6.3, 12.5
miconazole 6.3
micro-abrasion 4.16

Mitchell's trimmers 5.12
molars
    endodontic treatment 4.13
    furcation 3.4
    iatrogenic damage 4.5, 4.6, 4.7
mouthwash 3.2, 12.11
    following tooth extraction 5.4
    for plaque control 3.2
    for ulcers 6.2
mucocoele 7.5, 12.1
myofascial pain 5.9

N

nasopharyngeal airways 9.7
neck
    examination 1.4
    lumps 1.4
    swelling 1.4
necrotising ulcerative gingivitis 3.1
needlestick injuries 12.4
negligence 11.2
neurology
    causes of altered sensation 4.7
    cranial nerves 1.3
neutrophils 7.7
nifedipine 10.5
nursing caries 2.11
nystatin 6.3

O

occipito-mental radiograph 8.5
occlusal radiography 8.1
oculomotor nerve 1.3
odontogenic keratocyst 7.3
olfactory nerve 1.3
optic nerve 1.3
oral hygiene advice 3.1, 3.2, 5.4
orbital floor fracture 8.8
oropharyngeal airways 9.7

orthodontics 2.5, 2.6, 2.17
    gap closure 4.19
    upper orthodontic appliance 2.15

P

pain
    atypical facial 1.1, 10.4
    chest 12.9
    during jaw movement 5.9
    following tooth extraction 5.4
    toothache 3.3, 5.14
parallax technique 8.2
pathology request forms 7.1
pemphigoid 7.4
penicillamine 10.5
perforation, traumatic 4.6
periapical lesions, diagnosis 3.3
periapical radiography 8.1
pericoronitis 12.5
periodic acid-Schiff stain 7.7
periodontal disease 3.1, 3.2
periodontal examination 3.7
periodontal lesions
    diagnosis 3.3
    in pregnancy 3.8
    scoring and treatment 3.7
    see also specific conditions
periodontal probes 3.7
periodontitis 3.6
phenytoin 10.5
phlebotomy 9.4
plaque 3.1, 3.2
    control methods 3.1, 3.2
    scaling 3.9
polyps 4.12, 12.7
polyps *see* fibroepithelial polyps posts
posts 4.12
precancerous lesions 6.12
pregnancy 3.8
pregnancy epulis 3.8
prescriptions 10.4, 12.5
prilocaine 10.7

primary teeth
    avulsed 2.7
    retained 2.5
    vital pulpotomy 2.10
probes 3.7
prostheses *see* bridges; dentures
pulp
    Cvek pulpotomy 2.9
    damage to 2.7
    vitality testing 4.13
    vital pulpotomy 2.10
pulpal pocket 3.3
pulp chamber, perforation of 4.6
pulpotomy 2.9
pulse, taking the 9.5
pyogenic granuloma 3.8

amalgam 4.8
    composite 4.8
resuscitation 9.1
retruded jaw opening exercises 5.13
rheumatoid arthritis 10.5, 12.2
root canal treatment (RCT) 5.14
    accidental perforation 4.6
    broken file in canal 4.5
    filling in canal 4.7
    isolation methods for 4.14
    in primary teeth 2.10
roots
    displacement 8.11
    fracture 2.8
    furcation involvement 3.4
    periapical vs. periodontal lesions 3.3
rubber dams 4.14

R

radiography
    cephalometry 2.3
    dental panoramic tomography 8.7, 8.10
    filling in dental canal 4.7
    impacted canine teeth 2.5
    mandible 8.4, 8.10
    occipito-mental view 8.5
    orbits 8.8
    radiation protection 8.9
    rating 8.12
    skull anatomy 8.6
    techniques 8.1, 8.2, 8.3
rampant caries 2.11
RCT *see* root canal treatment
referral
    for infections 5.7
    for malignant ulcers 5.2
re-implantation 2.7, 2.13
    splints 2.12
restoration
    of crowns 4.11, 12.7
    materials 4.8
restorations

S

salbutamol 12.9
salivary glands
    mucocoele 7.5, 12.1
    tests of activity 6.5
    underactivity 6.4, 10.5
scaling 3.9
Schirmer's test 6.5
scintigraphy 6.5
scrubbing up 12.3
sealants 2.14
sedation 5.3, 5.6, 9.8
seizures 9.2, 12.9
sialography 6.5
side-effects of drugs 10.5
sight, testing 1.5
sinuses 5.8
Sjögren's syndrome 6.5
skull
    anatomy 8.6, 8.7
    cephalometry 2.3, 2.4
    fractures 8.4, 8.5, 8.8
smoking, advice on quitting 6.1

Snellen chart 1.5
sphygmomanometers 9.5
splints 2.7, 2.12
squamous-cell carcinoma 12.1
statistics 12.11
sterile procedures 12.3
steroids 6.2, 6.8, 12.2, 12.9
stomatitis, caused by dentures 4.3, 6.3
submandibular swellings 12.6
supernumerary teeth 2.6
surveying 4.15
sutures 5.10, 5.18
swanneck deformity 12.2
swellings *see* lumps
syncope (fainting) 9.1

T

temporomandibular joints (TMJs)
    dislocation 5.11
    examination 1.2
    jaw movement 1.2, 4.9, 5.13
tetracyclines 3.6, 4.16
thyroid gland 1.4
TMJ *see* temporomandibular joints
tomography
    computed 8.8
    dental panoramic 8.7, 8.10
toothache 3.3
toothbrushes 3.2
toothpaste 2.2, 3.2
toothpicks 3.2
traumatic injury
    avulsion of teeth 2.7, 2.13
    fractured teeth 2.8, 2.9, 12.7
    skull fractures 8.4, 8.5, 8.8
traumatic perforation 4.6
trigeminal nerve 1.3
trochlear nerve 1.3
tumours *see* cancer

U

ulcerative gingivitis
    acute 6.3
    necrotising 3.1
ulcers
    aphthous 6.2
    diagnosis 5.1, 7.4
    malignant 5.1, 5.2, 12.1
    see also stomatitis
ultrasonic scalers 3.9
unerupted teeth
    delayed eruption 2.5, 2.6
    radiographic localisation 8.2
upper orthodontic appliance 27

V

vagus nerve 1.3
veneers 4.11, 4.16
vestibulocochlear nerve 1.3
vicarious liability 11.2
vision, testing 1.5
vitality tests 3.3, 4.13
vital pulpotomy 2.10
vitamin C (diagnostic acronym) 12.8

W

Ward's buccal retractors 5.12
warfarin 5.16, 9.9
Warwick James elevators 5.12
wear, abnormal 4.4
wisdom teeth, extraction of 5.5

Z

zinc phosphate cement 4.1
zygoma, fracture 8.5

NOTES